The Ultimate Zer̲o̲ ̲P̲o̲i̲n̲t̲
Weight Loss Cookbook

*365 Days of Easy No Point Recipes for Fast Weight Loss and
Without Counting Calories*
Full Color Photos with 28-Day Meal Plan and Expert Advice

Table of Contents

Introduction

Welcome to a world where healthy eating and enjoyment go hand in hand. If you've struggled with weight loss programs that leave you feeling unsatisfied or diets that seem more like a punishment than a way of living, you're in the right place. The "0 Point Weight Loss Cookbook" is about transforming your relationship with food, making each meal a celebration of flavor without the guilt.

Welcome to a Healthier You

Imagine a day that begins with a delicious breakfast, continues with a satisfying lunch, includes a delightful snack, and concludes with a dinner that feels like a treat, yet all the while, you are losing weight and improving your health. That day can be every day. This cookbook isn't just about recipes—it's about giving you the tools to create a healthier lifestyle for yourself and your loved ones.

You might wonder how such a thing is possible. The secret lies in choosing the right ingredients and understanding how to use them to their full potential. Every choice in this book has been designed to optimize your health without compromising taste. From invigorating breakfasts to lush dinners, your meals will be as nutritious as they are delicious.

The Philosophy Behind Zero Point Foods

The concept of zero point foods is simple yet revolutionary. These are foods that you can eat without counting calories or points, foods that fill you up without weighing you down. Think of vegetables that burst with color and flavor, fruits that are as sweet as any dessert, and proteins that are both lean and savory. These ingredients are the backbone of the recipes in this book.

Why zero point foods? Because they are low in calories but high in fiber, water, and nutrients, they help you feel full longer and provide the energy you need to tackle your day. By building meals around these foods, you can eat until you are satisfied without overeating. This approach simplifies the often tedious task of tracking calories and aligns with a holistic view of health and wellness.

These zero point foods are not just a dietary choice; they are a lifestyle shift. They allow you to enjoy a range of textures and flavors—from crunchy and raw to soft and savory—without the stress of dietary restrictions. This freedom is transformative, enabling you to explore new culinary territories while knowing you are nourishing your body with every bite.

Embracing zero point foods means rethinking what it means to eat well. It's about changing your perception of portion sizes, understanding the nutritional value of your meals, and learning how to season and spice your dishes in ways that enhance their natural goodness without adding unnecessary calories. It's about making every meal an opportunity for nourishment and pleasure.

As you turn the pages of this cookbook, you'll discover that zero point foods are more than just ingredients—they are the building blocks of a vibrant, healthful life. With them, you will whip up hearty breakfasts that energize, lunches that fuel your afternoons, and dinners that satisfy. These meals will maintain your weight management goals and bring joy and abundance to your dining table.

The "0 Point Weight Loss Cookbook" aims to show you how easy and enjoyable healthy eating can be. No more feeling deprived or restricted; instead, you get to revel in the abundance that nature offers. This book will guide you through understanding and utilizing zero point foods to their fullest, ensuring that you can live a healthier, happier life without sacrificing the pleasures of eating well.

Get ready to transform the way you think about dieting. With "The 0 Point Weight Loss Cookbook," you'll learn how to make meals that are rich in nutrients and full of flavor, all while keeping your calorie intake in check. This isn't just a diet—it's a new way of life, a path to better health and greater satisfaction at the dining table. Let's begin this delicious adventure together, one recipe at a time.

How This Cookbook Can Change Your Life

Changing your diet can seem daunting, but this book is designed to ease that transition. You won't find strict rules or complicated meal plans here. Instead, you'll discover a new way to look at food and its preparation. With over 100 recipes divided across essential meal, including snacks and desserts, you have a wide array of options to choose from each day.

Each recipe in this book has been crafted not only for its taste but also for its health benefits, ensuring that you are nourished by every bite. Whether you are cooking for one or preparing a meal for a gathering, these dishes are designed to impress without stress.

Furthermore, the cookbook offers a 4-week Kickstart Meal Plan. This plan isn't just a list of meals but a guide to integrating zero point foods into your daily life effortlessly. It's structured to gradually introduce you to various dishes and ingredients, so by the end of the month, you'll be more than just acquainted with zero point cooking—you'll be in love with it.

You will learn not only how to cook these meals but also how to think creatively about ingredients and nutrition. As you flip through the pages, you'll find yourself gaining more than just cooking skills; you'll adopt a lifestyle that uplifts, energizes, and sustains.

This cookbook is more than a collection of recipes—it's a companion in your journey to better health. Each page is a step towards a more vibrant, healthier you, with guidance that is easy to follow and results that are easy to enjoy. Whether you are a seasoned chef or a novice in the kitchen, these recipes will bring the joy of eating back into your life, proving once and for all that healthy food can be fantastic food. Let's turn the page and start cooking up a storm of taste and wellness!

Chapter 1: Understanding 0 Point Weight Loss

What Are Zero Point Foods?

Zero Point Foods are at the heart of a revolutionary way to approach eating and weight loss. They consist of items that you can eat without needing to track calories, carbs, or fat grams. The idea is based on choosing foods that are low in calories but high in nutrients—foods that nourish your body without adding much to your daily caloric intake.

This concept typically includes a variety of fruits, vegetables, lean proteins, and certain whole grains. Imagine an array of colorful bell peppers, crisp apples, tender spinach, and robust chickpeas, all making up a diet that you don't have to measure or weigh. Zero Point Foods are not just about eating without guilt; they're about making smart, health-conscious choices that naturally complement your body's needs.

The appeal of Zero Point Foods lies in their ability to fill you up without filling you out. They are packed with fiber, water, vitamins, and minerals, which help to control hunger and boost satiety. This makes dieting less about restriction and more about making wise choices. It's a subtle shift in eating habits that encourages long-term health benefits and sustainable weight management.

Indeed, embracing Zero Point Foods can feel like unlocking a secret to effortless weight management. But it's no magic—it's science. These foods help stabilize blood sugar levels, reducing the highs and lows that can lead to overeating. They also enhance digestive health, ensuring that you absorb all the nutrients from the foods you consume while maintaining a healthy gut.

The high water content of many Zero Point Foods helps keep you hydrated and contributes to a feeling of fullness that can help curb unnecessary snacking. Hydration is often overlooked in discussions about dieting, but it's a crucial component of a healthy weight loss strategy. By integrating foods like cucumbers, strawberries, and tomatoes, which are over 90% water, you naturally enhance your hydration levels throughout the day.

Another fantastic aspect of Zero Point Foods is their versatility in cooking. You can steam, bake, grill, or sauté them, allowing for a multitude of preparation methods that can fit any taste preference and cooking skill level. The robust flavors and textures make meals exciting and satisfying. For instance, imagine grilling zucchini with a sprinkle of herbs for a delightful side dish, or blending frozen berries with Greek yogurt for a refreshing morning smoothie.

The strategy of Zero Point Foods supports meal creativity. With an emphasis on variety and flavor, these foods push you to experiment in the kitchen. They challenge you to think outside the box and discover new ways to enjoy healthy eating. Whether it's trying out different spices to enhance the natural flavors of a dish or mixing textures to create a satisfying meal, the possibilities are endless.

Moreover, the accessibility of Zero Point Foods means they are available in most grocery stores, making it easy for anyone to adopt this eating style. This accessibility supports the sustainable nature of the diet—it's not about exotic ingredients that are hard to find or expensive; it's about making the best of what's readily available.

This approach to dieting is not just a fad; it's a sustainable way to live a healthier life. It aligns with all that we know about nutrition and wellness, providing a practical and enjoyable way to eat well and lose weight without feeling deprived.

Benefits of the 0 Point Lifestyle

Adopting a 0 Point Lifestyle can truly transform your approach to eating and weight loss. The benefits are manifold and affect not just your physical health but your mental well-being and lifestyle flexibility.

Simplified Dieting

The beauty of the 0 Point system is its simplicity. It eradicates the need for meticulous calorie counting or tracking every single bite you eat. This approach liberates you from the daily grind of monitoring every calorie, which can be both tiresome and demoralizing. Instead, you can enjoy unlimited amounts of Zero Point Foods, which significantly relieves the psychological burden often associated with dieting. This simplicity makes it far easier to stick to your health and wellness goals, as the process becomes more about enjoying what you eat rather than restricting yourself.

Increased Nutrient Intake

When your diet focuses on nutrient-dense foods, you naturally enhance the quality of your meals. This isn't just about eating less—it's about nourishing your body more effectively. The high levels of vitamins, minerals, and fiber in Zero Point Foods can lead to markedly improved health outcomes. You might notice better digestion thanks to the increased fiber, more stable blood sugar levels from eating whole, unprocessed foods, and a significant boost in energy, all of which are vital components of a healthy lifestyle. This increase in nutrient intake supports bodily functions and can contribute to long-term health and vitality.

Natural Portion Control

One of the most practical benefits of the 0 Point Lifestyle is natural portion control. Zero Point Foods are typically high in fiber, which helps you feel fuller sooner and for a longer period.

This means you are likely to eat less naturally, without feeling restricted or unsatisfied. Over time, this can lead to weight loss that doesn't require constant oversight or micro-management of your diet. It's about feeling full and content, not deprived and hungry, which can make all the difference in how sustainable your eating habits are.

Flexible and Sustainable

The flexibility of the 0 Point Lifestyle is another significant benefit. It is not a rigid diet with harsh rules but a flexible eating plan that can easily adapt to different tastes and living situations. Whether you are cooking at home, enjoying a meal out, or even traveling, you can find options that fit within the Zero Point framework. This adaptability makes it more likely that you can stick with this eating style over the long haul, integrating it into your life regardless of the situation. It accommodates changes in your routine or lifestyle, ensuring that healthy eating is always accessible.

Promotes Healthy Habits

Perhaps most importantly, the 0 Point Lifestyle fosters the development of healthy habits that extend beyond mere dieting. It encourages you to make healthier food choices consistently, not just during a diet phase but as a permanent way of living. This lifestyle shift is about embracing foods that benefit your body, learning to love what is good for you, and creating habits that will maintain both your health and your well-being into the future.

This approach to eating and wellness goes beyond typical diet benefits. It helps build a relationship with food that is based on appreciation and understanding rather than restriction and counting. By focusing on what you can eat freely and without guilt, the 0 Point Lifestyle helps recalibrate your mindset about food. It shifts the focus from fearing food to embracing it as a source of nourishment and enjoyment.

Moreover, this lifestyle supports your mental health by reducing diet-related stress and anxiety. It fosters a positive outlook where food is not seen as the enemy but as a friend that supports your health goals. The absence of strict rules and the presence of freedom in food choices can significantly increase your satisfaction with your diet, which is crucial for mental and emotional well-being.

The 0 Point Lifestyle is not just a way to lose weight. It simplifies eating, enriches your diet with nutrients, provides flexibility, and promotes a sustainable approach to health that can adapt to any lifestyle. Most importantly, it helps cultivate a positive mindset toward eating, focusing on abundance and satisfaction rather than limitations and deprivation. This holistic approach is why so many find lasting success and fulfillment in adopting the 0 Point way of living.

Common Myths Debunked

When it comes to any diet or lifestyle change, misconceptions can arise, and the 0 Point Lifestyle is no exception. Let's clear up some common myths:

Myth 1: You can eat as much as you want.

While it's true that Zero Point Foods are low in calories, they should still be eaten in moderation. The key is to listen to your body's hunger cues and eat until you feel satisfied, not stuffed. It's easy to assume that because something is labeled as "zero points," it means you can consume it in unlimited quantities. However, true dietary balance and health come from moderation and variety. Overeating, even low-calorie foods, can still lead to digestive discomfort and may not provide the balance of nutrients that your body needs.

Myth 2: Zero Point Foods are enough for a balanced diet.

Although Zero Point Foods are healthy, they are just one part of a balanced diet. Including a variety of other foods ensures you receive a complete range of nutrients. Healthy fats, for instance, are crucial for vitamin absorption and brain health, while proteins are essential for muscle repair and growth. Both are typically not classified as zero points but are vital for overall health. Thus, it's essential to integrate a spectrum of nutritional options in your meals to maintain health and well-being.

Myth 3: The 0 Point Lifestyle is just another fad diet.

Unlike many fad diets that come and go, the principles underlying the 0 Point approach are based on sound nutritional advice—eat more fruits, vegetables, and lean proteins, and fewer high-calorie foods. This advice stands the test of time for maintaining a healthy weight and preventing disease. The 0 Point Lifestyle isn't about quick fixes or severe restrictions that are unsustainable in the long term; it's about learning to make healthier food choices that you can continue throughout your life.

Myth 4: Zero Point Foods are bland and boring.

This could not be further from the truth! With the right recipes and cooking techniques, Zero Point Foods can be transformed into delicious meals that satisfy even the most discerning palate. The diversity of foods within this category means there are endless possibilities for creative, flavorful dishes. Fresh herbs, spices, and simple culinary techniques can elevate these ingredients into exciting and enjoyable meals. Think about grilling stone fruit for a caramelized dessert, using aromatic spices to enhance a vegetable stew, or combining fresh vegetables with herbs for a vibrant salad. The options are limitless and anything but boring.

Myth 5: Adopting a 0 Point Lifestyle is too difficult and restrictive.

Some might think that following a diet based around Zero Point Foods restricts their culinary options, but this is actually a liberating way to eat. This lifestyle promotes exploring a wide range of foods that perhaps weren't previously part of your diet. It encourages you to experiment with new recipes and ingredients, broadening your culinary repertoire. Furthermore, because you aren't counting calories, you spend less time worrying about the numbers and more time enjoying food.

Myth 6: You won't get enough protein on the 0 Point Lifestyle.

It's a common concern that diets focusing primarily on fruits and vegetables fail to provide adequate protein. However, many Zero Point Foods are rich in protein, such as legumes, certain seafood, and low-fat dairy products. These can be incorporated into your diet to meet your protein needs without compromising the diet's principles. Combining different plant-based proteins can also provide all the essential amino acids your body requires.

Myth 7: The diet doesn't support social eating or dining out.

People often worry that following specific diets will hinder their social lives or dining out experiences. However, the 0 Point Lifestyle is versatile enough to adapt to restaurant menus and social settings. Many restaurants offer dishes that feature plenty of fruits, vegetables, and lean proteins, and learning how to make smart choices while dining out is an integral part of this lifestyle. Moreover, it provides an opportunity to educate friends and family about healthier eating in a social context, perhaps even influencing their choices for the better.

Chapter 2: Setting Up Your Zero Point Kitchen

Creating a kitchen that supports your 0 Point Lifestyle is not just about having the right foods at hand; it's about setting up an environment that encourages healthy eating and simplifies the process of meal preparation. This chapter will guide you through selecting essential tools and utensils, stocking your pantry with Zero Point staples, and keeping your kitchen organized to support your new way of eating.

Essential Cooking Tools and Utensils

Ensuring your kitchen is well-equipped is foundational to the success of any diet plan, especially one centered on the Zero Point philosophy. This means having the right tools that not only make meal preparation easier but also more enjoyable.

Quality Knives

Good quality knives transform kitchen time from chore to delight. You'll want a versatile chef's knife that can handle everything from slicing meats to dicing vegetables, a paring knife for the more delicate tasks such as peeling fruits or finely chopping garlic, and a serrated knife that can slice through breads and tomatoes with ease. Sharp and well-balanced, these knives ensure that your prep work is efficient and precise.

Cutting Boards

To maintain hygiene and prevent cross-contamination, keep at least two cutting boards in your kitchen: one for fresh produce and the other for raw meats, if they are part of your diet. Opt for bamboo or wooden boards for produce; they are durable and less likely to dull your knives compared to plastic boards.

Blenders and Food Processors

For making smoothies, purees, or soups, a high-powered blender is indispensable. It can also crush ice and blend frozen fruits for quick sorbets or frozen yogurt. A food processor, on the other hand, is invaluable for more labor-intensive tasks like chopping large quantities of vegetables, making doughs, or grinding nuts and seeds. These tools are essential for anyone looking to simplify complex recipes and reduce manual prep time.

Non-Stick Cookware

A variety of non-stick cookware in your cabinet means you're always prepared, whether you're cooking a single egg or a large pot of stew. Non-stick surfaces are crucial for cooking with minimal oil and ensure easy clean-up, which can be a huge time-saver in the kitchen.

Measuring Cups and Spoons

When you are adjusting to how much of certain foods you should consume, accurate measuring tools are vital. They help ensure you are following recipes correctly, which is important not just for taste but for maintaining the nutritional integrity of your meals. Consistency is vital in cooking, and proper measurements lead to consistent results.

Mixing Bowls

A set of mixing bowls in various sizes is fundamental for any kitchen. These bowls are perfect for mixing together salad ingredients, combining marinades, or just holding your prepped ingredients before cooking. Having bowls that nest within each other can save space and provide options for any meal size, from single servings to family-sized dishes.

Kitchen Scales

A reliable kitchen scale is a must for those precise recipes where every gram counts. It's particularly helpful for maintaining portion control, which is essential in a Zero Point diet. Digital scales offer an easy and accurate way to measure ingredients, which helps keep your meals consistent with your dietary goals.

Colanders and Sieves

Colanders and sieves are necessary tools for washing vegetables and fruits or for draining cooked foods like pasta and beans. They are also useful for sifting dry ingredients for baking, ensuring smoother textures in your dishes.

Silicone Utensils

Silicone utensils, such as spatulas, spoons, and ladles, are gentle on non-stick surfaces and withstand high temperatures. Their flexibility and non-stick properties make them ideal for scraping, stirring, and spreading, ensuring you get every last bit of your preparation without damaging your cookware.

Peeler and Grater

A sharp peeler can save you time and effort in skinning fruits and vegetables. A robust grater is equally essential for adding a zest of freshness to your dishes, whether it's chocolate over a dessert or Parmesan on your pasta.

Citrus Juicer

A hand-held citrus juicer extracts maximum juice from lemons, limes, and oranges, which can enhance the flavor of a dish or simply provide a fresh squeeze for your morning water or tea. It's a simple tool that adds a punch of flavor with minimal effort.

With these tools and utensils, your kitchen will be well-prepared to handle the demands of the Zero Point Lifestyle. Each item plays a critical role in making your cooking process smoother and more efficient, contributing to a diet that feels less like a chore and more like a part of your daily enjoyment. As you equip your kitchen, you're not just investing in tools but in your health and well-being, making every meal an opportunity to nourish your body while delighting your palate.

Tips for Maintaining an Organized Kitchen

An organized kitchen is crucial for making your diet plan manageable and enjoyable. It transforms cooking from a chore into a delightful part of your day. Maintaining an orderly kitchen requires a bit of planning and regular upkeep, but the payoff is a smoother, more efficient cooking experience.

Organize by Zone

Dividing your kitchen into zones based on activities—storing, prepping, cooking, and cleaning—creates an efficient workspace. Arrange your kitchen so that everything you need for each task is within easy reach. For example, keep all your pots, pans, and cooking utensils near the stove. Place your cutting boards, knives, and other prep tools in a dedicated prep area. This zoning not only streamlines your cooking process but also helps in maintaining cleanliness and order.

Use Clear Containers

Using clear containers for storage is one of the simplest yet most effective organizational tactics. These containers allow you to see what's inside without opening them, which not only saves time but also reduces the risk of using expired or spoiled ingredients. Label each container clearly with the contents and expiration date to further streamline your kitchen management. This practice is beneficial for bulk items like grains, nuts, and spices, which can otherwise become cluttered and difficult to manage.

Regularly Clean and Declutter

Regular maintenance is key to an organized kitchen. Set a schedule to clean out your refrigerator and pantry. Remove everything, dispose of expired or spoiled items, and wipe down all surfaces before putting items back. This routine not only ensures cleanliness but also helps you keep an inventory of your stock to avoid over-purchasing or wasting food. Regular decluttering also applies to your utensils, gadgets, and cookware. If you find you haven't used an item in a year, consider donating it to clear space and reduce clutter.

Plan Your Space

If possible, dedicate a small area in your kitchen for meal planning and recipe review. This could be a small desk area where you keep your cookbooks, notepads, pens, and nutritional information, or even just a corner of your kitchen counter with a dedicated notebook and pen. Having a specific spot for planning makes it more likely that you will stick to your meal plans because it integrates the planning process into your daily kitchen use.

Streamline Your Cooking Tools

Evaluate your cooking tools and appliances. Keep only those that serve multiple purposes or are essential to your daily cooking. This not only frees up space but also reduces the time you spend searching for the right tool. For example, a high-quality food processor can often do the work of several gadgets like a blender, mixer, and chopper.

Maximize Vertical Space

Utilize vertical spaces with hanging pots and utensil racks, magnetic knife strips, and overhead cabinets. This not only saves counter space but also puts your tools in easy reach. Adjustable shelves in cabinets allow you to customize storage according to your needs, making it easier to store tall appliances or stackable items.

Invest in Quality Storage Solutions

Invest in durable, high-quality storage solutions that can handle the wear and tear of kitchen use. Drawer dividers, spice racks, and under-shelf baskets can dramatically increase your storage capacity and help keep your countertops clear.

Create a System That Works for You

Everyone's cooking style and kitchen layout are different, so it's important to create an organizational system that suits your personal needs. Think about the steps you take when you cook and organize your kitchen to complement this flow. This personalized approach means you'll be more likely to maintain the organization because it naturally fits into your daily routine.

By setting up your kitchen with clear zones, maintaining regular cleaning routines, and using effective storage solutions, you create an environment that supports your Zero Point Lifestyle. This organized space not only makes cooking more enjoyable but also helps you stay committed to your healthy eating goals. With everything in its place, you can focus more on creating delicious, healthy meals and less on managing chaos, making your kitchen a haven of creativity and health.

Chapter 3: Smart Shopping

Shopping smartly is foundational to maintaining a healthy diet, especially when you are following a Zero Point Lifestyle. This chapter is dedicated to teaching you how to navigate the supermarket to find the best foods for your health and budget. We will cover how to choose the right foods, understand food labels, and share some tips to stretch your food budget without sacrificing quality.

Choosing the Right Foods at the Supermarket

When you shop at the supermarket, your goal should be to fill your cart with foods that support your Zero Point Lifestyle—foods that are nutritious, filling, and free from unnecessary additives.

Start with Fresh Produce

The produce section is typically the first area you enter in a supermarket. This is where you should spend a good portion of your shopping time. Look for a variety of colors in fruits and vegetables, as these colors represent different nutrients and antioxidants. Fresh produce not only adds essential vitamins and minerals to your diet but also increases your intake of fiber, which is crucial for feeling full and satisfied without adding a lot of calories.

Lean Proteins

Next, move to the protein section. Opt for lean meats like chicken breast, turkey, and lean cuts of beef or pork. Fish is also a great choice, particularly fatty types like salmon, which are high in omega-3 fatty acids. If you are vegetarian or vegan, look for plant-based proteins such as tofu, tempeh, and a variety of beans and legumes that can be excellent substitutes for animal protein.

Whole Grains

Incorporate whole grains into your diet instead of refined grains. Look for whole grain breads, pastas, and cereals that list a whole grain as the first ingredient. Whole grains provide more nutrients and fiber than their refined counterparts, which helps with digestion and prolongs the feeling of fullness.

Dairy or Alternatives

Choose low-fat dairy products or plant-based alternatives. Pay attention to the sugar content in yogurt and milk alternatives, as these can often contain added sugars. Opting for unsweetened or plain versions allows you to control the amount of sugar you consume.

Understanding Food Labels

Reading food labels is crucial to making informed choices about the foods you eat. Labels can tell you a lot about the nutritional value of a product, helping you to avoid those that are high in sugars, fats, and sodium.

Check Serving Sizes

Begin by looking at the serving size and the number of servings per container. This information will help you assess how much you are actually consuming. Sometimes, packages that appear to be single servings are actually two or more.

Look at Nutritional Content

Examine the calories and nutrients to determine how this fits into your daily nutritional goals. Focus on dietary fiber, protein, vitamins, and minerals. Higher fiber and protein content can be particularly beneficial as they help promote satiety and muscle repair.

Identify Added Sugars and Sodium

Avoid foods high in added sugars and sodium. The nutritional label will list these, and they are often found in higher quantities in processed foods. Opting for items with no added sugars and low sodium can significantly impact your health.

Understand Ingredient Lists

The ingredients list should be short and contain items that you recognize. Ingredients are listed in order of quantity, so those at the beginning of the list make up the bulk of the food. Avoid products with long lists of unrecognizable ingredients, as these are often highly processed.

Budget Tips for Healthy Eating

Eating healthily doesn't have to break the bank. With a few strategies, you can eat well, even on a tight budget.

Plan Your Meals

Planning your meals for the week ahead can save money and reduce food waste. Check what you already have at home before shopping and build your meal plans around those ingredients. Buy only what you need for the planned meals.

Buy in Bulk

Purchasing staple items like rice, pasta, and beans in bulk can save money in the long run. These items have a long shelf life when stored properly and can be used in a variety of meals.

Shop Seasonally

Fruits and vegetables are usually less expensive when they are in season. They are also at their peak flavor and nutritional content. Learn what produce is in season and plan your meals accordingly.

Use Coupons and Rewards

Take advantage of any coupons, sales, and store reward cards. Many supermarkets offer loyalty programs that can provide significant savings over time.

Cook at Home

Preparing your meals at home can be much cheaper than eating out. Home-cooked meals are also likely to be healthier and better portion-controlled.

By shopping smartly, reading food labels carefully, and applying budget-friendly tips, you can enjoy a nutritious diet that supports your Zero Point Lifestyle without stressing your wallet. This approach not only fosters better physical health but also ensures you are entirely in control of what you eat by making conscious choices that are good for you and your budget.

Chapter 4: The Complete List of Zero Point Foods

In the Zero Point Lifestyle, embracing a wide array of vegetables and fruits is key to enjoying a nutritious, satisfying diet without the need to meticulously count calories.

Vegetables

Vegetables are pivotal in any nutritious diet, particularly under the Zero Point plan, where they are celebrated for their low calorie yet high-nutrient content. Here are the types of vegetables you can enjoy abundantly:

Leafy Greens

- **Spinach**: Rich in iron and vitamins A, C, and K, spinach is versatile for salads and cooked dishes.
- **Kale**: Packed with nutrients, kale can be used in smoothies or sautéed as a side.
- **Arugula**: With its peppery flavor, arugula is great in salads or as a pizza topping.
- **Romaine Lettuce**: Crisp and refreshing, perfect for salads and wraps.

Cruciferous Vegetables

- **Broccoli**: High in fiber and vitamins C and K, it can be eaten raw or cooked.
- **Cauliflower**: Great for roasting or as a mashed potato substitute.
- **Brussels Sprouts**: Best roasted or steamed, these offer a nutty flavor.
- **Cabbage**: Versatile for slaws or cooked into stews and soups.

Alliums

- **Onions**: A base for many dishes, providing depth and sweetness when cooked.
- **Garlic**: Used in almost every cuisine in the world, it's essential for flavoring.
- **Leeks**: Milder than onions, excellent in pies and soups.
- **Shallots**: Combine the flavors of onions and garlic, enhancing both cooked and raw dishes.

Additional Vegetables

- **Bell Peppers**: Available in various colors, adding sweetness and crunch.
- **Zucchini**: Ideal for grilling, stir-fries, or making zucchini noodles.
- **Summer Squash**: Similar to zucchini, great for sautéing or baking.
- **Eggplants**: Absorb flavors well, perfect for dishes like ratatouille or baba ganoush.
- **Mushrooms**: Offer a meaty texture, suitable for vegetarian dishes.
- **Asparagus**: Excellent steamed, grilled, or in omelets.

- **Snap Peas**: Crunchy and sweet, ideal for snacking or quick stir-fries.
- **Green Beans**: Versatile for side dishes, whether steamed, sautéed, or in casseroles.
- **Tomatoes**: Fresh or cooked, they are a staple in salads, sauces, and sandwiches.
- **Cucumbers**: Refreshing in salads or as a garnish for drinks.
- **Celery**: Adds a crisp texture and flavor to salads and snacks.
- **Carrots**: Sweet and crunchy, good for snacking, roasting, or in stews.

Fruits

Fruits are celebrated not only for their natural sweetness and flavor but also for their health benefits, as they provide essential vitamins, minerals, and fiber. Here's a comprehensive list of Zero Point fruits:

Berries

- **Strawberries**: Enjoy them fresh, in salads, or desserts.
- **Blueberries**: Perfect for oatmeal, yogurt, or by themselves.
- **Raspberries**: Great in desserts or as a fresh snack.
- **Blackberries**: Delicious whether eaten alone or stirred into a fruit salad.

Citrus Fruits

- **Oranges**: Juicy and sweet, ideal for snacking or juicing.
- **Grapefruits**: A bit tart, perfect for breakfast or in fruit salads.
- **Lemons**: Add zest and brightness to drinks and dishes.
- **Limes**: Key for adding a tangy flavor to beverages and meals.

Stone Fruits

- **Peaches**: Juicy and sweet, perfect for eating fresh or in desserts.
- **Nectarines**: Similar to peaches, but with a smoother skin.
- **Plums**: Sweet and tart, suitable for eating fresh or in jams.
- **Cherries**: Enjoyable fresh, or use them in pies and preserves.

Other Fruits

- **Apples**: Versatile for eating raw, baked, or stewed.
- **Pears**: Sweet and juicy, great for snacking or baking.
- **Bananas**: Energy-rich, ideal for breakfast or as a snack.
- **Melons**: Watermelon, cantaloupe, and honeydew are refreshing, especially when chilled.
- **Kiwi**: Offers a tropical flavor and plenty of vitamin C.
- **Pineapple**: Sweet and tangy, perfect for fruit salads or grilled.

Proteins

Proteins are crucial for muscle repair, growth, and overall satiety, making them a vital component of any nutritious diet. Here's an expanded list of protein sources suitable for Zero Point eating:

- **Chicken Breast**: Skinless and versatile for a variety of dishes.
- **Turkey Breast**: Low in fat and high in protein, ideal for roasting or grilling.
- **Salmon and Trout**: Rich in omega-3 fatty acids, perfect for heart health.
- **Haddock**: Light and flaky, suitable for baking or broiling.
- **Shrimp and Lobster**: Excellent sources of protein, great for seafood dishes.
- **Lean Cuts of Beef**: Such as sirloin or tenderloin, best cooked without added fat.
- **Pork Tenderloin**: Another lean option that's flavorful when roasted or grilled.
- **Egg Whites**: High in protein and versatile in omelets or mixed with whole eggs for a lighter option.

Whole Grains

Whole grains provide necessary fiber, which helps with digestion and maintains steady blood sugar levels, essential for a balanced diet:

- **Quinoa**: A complete protein, making it a staple in any diet.
- **Oats**: Known for their cholesterol-lowering effects.
- **Barley**: Nutritious and filling, ideal for soups and stews.
- **Farro**: Has a chewy texture and nutty flavor, perfect for salads and side dishes.
- **Bulgur Wheat**: Quick to prepare and a traditional ingredient in tabbouleh and other Middle Eastern dishes.

Legumes

Legumes are not only a fantastic source of plant-based protein and fiber but also enhance meal satiety and diversity:

- **Black Beans, Kidney Beans, and Chickpeas**: Nutritious and versatile, perfect for salads, soups, and as main dishes.
- **Lentils**: Available in various colors, quick to cook, and packed with nutrients.
- **Pinto Beans**: A staple in Mexican cuisine, excellent for refried beans or in chili.
- **Navy Beans**: Mild and creamy, great in soups or baked beans.
- **Mung Beans**: Often used in Asian recipes, they are adaptable for salads, curries, and soups.

Herbs and Spices

Herbs and spices are pivotal in enhancing the flavor of dishes without adding any calories, making them invaluable in the Zero Point kitchen. They not only improve taste but also contribute health benefits, making your meals both delicious and nutritious.

Herbs

Herbs bring fresh, aromatic flavors to any dish, making them a staple in kitchens around the world:

- **Basil**: Adds a sweet and slightly peppery flavor, perfect in Italian dishes like pesto or tomato-based sauces.
- **Cilantro**: Known for its lively, citrus-like taste, it is essential in Mexican and Asian cuisines.
- **Parsley**: Offers a mild, slightly bitter taste that complements a wide array of dishes, from soups to salads.
- **Mint**: Refreshing and cool, ideal for drinks, salads, or Middle Eastern dishes.
- **Rosemary**: With its woody fragrance, it's fantastic in roasts and Mediterranean cooking.
- **Thyme**: Subtle and slightly dry, it's a great addition to soups, stews, and poultry dishes.
- **Oregano**: A robust herb with a peppery bite, commonly used in Greek and Italian cuisines.
- **Dill**: Delicate and with a sweet taste that pairs well with fish and comes through in pickling.

Spices

Spices offer a range of flavors from sweet to smoky to hot, and many come with added health benefits:

- **Turmeric**: Known for its anti-inflammatory properties, it has a warm, bitter taste and gives curry its yellow color.
- **Cinnamon**: Sweet and woody, it's used in both sweet and savory dishes and is beneficial for blood sugar regulation.
- **Paprika**: Adds vibrant color and a sweet-to-smoky flavor, perfect for meats and stews.
- **Cumin**: Earthy and aromatic, essential in Middle Eastern, Indian, and Mexican cuisines.
- **Coriander**: Offers a citrus-like flavor when ground and is particularly good in spice mixes and curries.
- **Cardamom**: Sweet and spicy, used in Scandinavian and Middle Eastern baking and desserts.
- **Cayenne Pepper**: Brings heat and intensity to dishes, great in Cajun and Mexican recipes.

Vinegars and Mustards

These ingredients are crucial for adding piquant flavors to dishes without the addition of sugar or significant fats, making them perfect for dressing and marinades in a Zero Point setting.

Vinegars

Vinegars not only enhance the flavors in a dish but can also have health benefits:

- **Apple Cider Vinegar**: Often used in dressings, marinades, or even for its potential health benefits, including improved digestion and blood sugar control.
- **Balsamic Vinegar**: Sweet and tart, it can elevate salads, grilled vegetables, and even fresh fruits.
- **Red Wine Vinegar**: Bold and tangy, ideal for dressings and enhancing meat dishes.
- **Rice Vinegar**: Mild and slightly sweet, commonly used in Asian dishes, especially sushi and marinades.

Mustards

Mustards add a sharp, tangy depth to dishes, making them a flavorful addition without the need for calories:

- **Dijon Mustard**: Smooth and sharp, perfect for emulsifying dressings or as a rub for meats.
- **Whole Grain Mustard**: Adds texture and a robust flavor to vinaigrettes or as an accompaniment to cheese and meats.
- **Yellow Mustard**: Mild and versatile, commonly used in sandwiches, dressings, and classic American recipes.

Incorporating these Zero Point Foods into your meals ensures that your diet is not only aligned with your weight management goals but also varied and rich in nutrients. This approach allows for creativity in the kitchen, letting you enjoy a variety of flavorful meals that support both your health and culinary enjoyment.

Chapter 5: Understanding Portions and Satiety

Understanding how to manage portions and enhance satiety is fundamental in any nutritious diet, especially for those following a Zero Point lifestyle where the focus is on feeling full and satisfied without overeating. This chapter will delve into the art and science of portion control, explore foods that maximize fullness, and discuss how to balance your plate to achieve optimal satiety.

How to Measure Portions Accurately

Measuring portions accurately is essential to maintaining a healthy diet and ensuring you are consuming the right amount of food for your energy needs. It's about understanding the difference between a serving size, which is a measured amount of food, and a portion, which is the amount you choose to eat. Here are some practical tips to help you measure portions accurately:

Use Measuring Tools

Invest in a set of measuring cups, spoons, and a kitchen scale. These tools will help you follow recipes accurately and control portion sizes, especially for dense foods like grains and proteins, where it's easy to overeat.

Visual Comparisons

In situations where you can't measure food, visual comparisons can be a handy guide. For instance, a serving of cooked meat should be about the size of a deck of cards, a half-cup of pasta resembles a tennis ball, and an ounce of cheese looks like a pair of dice. Using these visual aids helps prevent portion distortion—a common issue where estimated portion sizes gradually increase over time.

Check Packaging

Food packaging often includes serving size information. Using the serving size listed on the package as a guide can help you determine how much of that food integrates into a balanced meal.

Foods That Maximize Fullness

To enhance satiety and avoid overeating, include foods in your diet that are known to promote a feeling of fullness. Foods that are high in protein, fiber, and water content are especially effective at keeping you satisfied between meals.

High-Fiber Foods

Foods like fruits, vegetables, whole grains, and legumes contain significant amounts of dietary fiber, which slows digestion and prolongs the feeling of fullness. For example, oatmeal for breakfast can help you feel full well into your day.

Protein-Rich Foods

Proteins are particularly effective at inducing satiety. Including a protein source in each meal and snack can help regulate hunger hormones and keep you feeling satisfied. Lean meats, fish, eggs, dairy products, and plant-based proteins like beans and lentils are excellent choices.

High-Water Content Foods

Fruits and vegetables like watermelon, cucumbers, oranges, and celery have high water content, which helps fill you up with fewer calories. Incorporating these into meals or having them as snacks can significantly enhance satiety.

Balancing Your Plate for Optimal Satiety

Balancing your plate with the right proportions of macronutrients (proteins, fats, and carbohydrates) and including plenty of fiber-rich foods are key to achieving and maintaining lasting fullness.

The Half-Plate Rule

A useful method to ensure a balanced meal is the half-plate rule: fill half of your plate with vegetables and fruits, a quarter with lean protein, and the remaining quarter with whole grains or another complex carbohydrate. This balance not only ensures a nutrient-rich meal but also helps manage calorie intake while maximizing satiety.

Include Healthy Fats

While fats are more calorie-dense, they are also crucial for satiety. Including a small amount of healthy fat, such as olive oil, nuts, or avocados, can prolong the feeling of fullness and enhance meal satisfaction.

Regular, Balanced Meals

Eating at regular intervals throughout the day ensures that your body receives a constant supply of nutrients, keeping hunger at bay and energy levels stable. Skipping meals can lead to overeating later, so it's important to include balanced meals and snacks as part of your daily routine.

By understanding how to accurately measure food portions, incorporating foods that enhance satiety, and balancing your plate, you can enjoy satisfying meals that support your health goals without the need to count every calorie. This approach to eating encourages a healthy relationship with food, where dieting shifts from restriction to enjoyment, allowing you to achieve both fullness and nutritional balance.

Chapter 6: Breakfast Delights

Sunrise Smoothie Bowl

Servings: 2

Prep Time: 10 minutes

Cook Time: 0 minutes

Ingredients:

- 2 cups frozen mango chunks (330g)
- 1 banana (120g)
- 1 cup unsweetened almond milk (240ml)
- 1/2 teaspoon ground turmeric (2g)
- 2 tablespoons chia seeds (20g)
- 1/2 cup sliced strawberries (75g)
- 2 tablespoons unsweetened coconut flakes (10g)
- 2 tablespoons sliced almonds (20g)

Instructions:

1. Combine frozen mango, banana, almond milk, and turmeric in a blender. Blend until smooth.
2. Pour the mixture into two bowls and evenly top with chia seeds, strawberries, coconut flakes, and almonds.
3. Serve immediately and enjoy the tropical flavors.

Kcal: 310 per serving, Cho: 47g, Fat: 12g, Na: 60mg, Pro: 6g

Berry Blast Overnight Oats

Servings: 2

Prep Time: 5 minutes

Cook Time: 0 minutes (refrigerate overnight)

Ingredients:

- 1 cup rolled oats (90g)
- 1 cup unsweetened almond milk (240ml)
- 2/3 cup Greek yogurt (low-fat) (160g)
- 1/4 teaspoon liquid stevia (or to taste)
- 1 cup mixed berries (raspberries, blueberries) (140g)

- 2 tablespoons ground flaxseed (14g)

Instructions:

1. In a medium bowl, mix rolled oats, almond milk, Greek yogurt, and stevia.
2. Gently fold in the mixed berries and sprinkle ground flaxseed on top.
3. Cover and refrigerate overnight.
4. Stir before eating and, if desired, top with additional berries.

Kcal: 315 per serving, Cho: 48g, Fat: 8g, Na: 55mg, Pro: 12g

Spinach and Mushroom Egg Muffins

Servings: 2 (6 muffins total, 3 per serving)

Prep Time: 10 minutes

Cook Time: 20 minutes

Ingredients:

- 8 large eggs (400g)
- 2 cups fresh spinach, chopped (60g)
- 1 cup diced mushrooms (150g)
- 1/2 cup diced red bell pepper (75g)
- 1/2 cup low-fat milk (120ml)
- Salt and pepper to taste

Instructions:

1. Preheat the oven to 350°F (177°C) and grease a muffin tin with non-stick spray.
2. Whisk eggs and milk together in a bowl. Season with salt and pepper.
3. Stir in the chopped spinach, mushrooms, and red bell pepper.
4. Evenly divide the mixture among the muffin cups.
5. Bake in the preheated oven for 20 minutes or until the muffins are set and lightly golden on top.
6. Allow to cool for a few minutes before removing from the muffin tin.

Kcal: 70 per muffin, Cho: 2g, Fat: 4g, Na: 125mg, Pro: 6g

Sweet Potato and Kale Hash

Servings: 2

Prep Time: 10 minutes

Cook Time: 15 minutes

Ingredients:

- 2 medium sweet potatoes, peeled and diced (400g)
- 2 cups chopped kale (134g)
- 1 red onion, diced (150g)
- 4 cloves garlic, minced (12g)
- 4 tablespoons olive oil (60ml)
- Salt and pepper to taste

Instructions:

1. Heat olive oil in a large skillet over medium heat.
2. Add diced sweet potatoes and cook for about 10 minutes, stirring occasionally, until nearly tender.
3. Add red onion and garlic to the skillet. Cook for another 3 minutes.
4. Stir in the chopped kale and cook until the kale is wilted and the sweet potatoes are tender, about 2 minutes.
5. Season with salt and pepper to taste and serve hot.

Kcal: 250 per serving, Cho: 27g, Fat: 14g, Na: 70mg, Pro: 4g

Cinnamon Apple Yogurt Parfait

Servings: 2

Prep Time: 5 minutes

Cook Time: 0 minutes

Ingredients:

- 2 cups low-fat Greek yogurt (490g)
- 2 small apples, diced (200g)
- 1 teaspoon ground cinnamon (2g)
- 1/4 teaspoon liquid stevia (or to taste)
- 4 tablespoons granola (no added sugar) (30g)

Instructions:

1. In two serving glasses, layer one cup of Greek yogurt at the bottom of each.
2. Combine diced apple with cinnamon and layer half over the yogurt in each glass.
3. Drizzle liquid stevia over the apples in each glass. Adjust the amount to match your sweetness preference, as stevia's sweetness can vary.
4. Repeat the layers with the remaining yogurt, apple, and stevia.
5. Top each parfait with 2 tablespoons of granola just before serving to maintain crunch.

Kcal: 315 per serving, Cho: 44g, Fat: 5g, Na: 85mg, Pro: 20g

Savory Oatmeal with Avocado

Servings: 2

Prep Time: 5 minutes

Cook Time: 10 minutes

Ingredients:

- 1 cup rolled oats (90g)
- 2 cups water (480ml)
- 1/2 teaspoon salt (3g)
- 1 avocado, diced (200g)
- 1/4 cup chopped fresh cilantro (4g)
- 1 tablespoon lime juice (15ml)
- 1 small jalapeño, seeded and minced (14g)
- 2 tablespoons chopped green onions (30g)

Instructions:

1. In a small saucepan, bring water and salt to a boil. Add oats and reduce heat to a simmer. Cook, stirring occasionally, until the oats are tender, about 5 minutes.
2. Remove from heat and let sit for 2 minutes to thicken.
3. Stir in the lime juice, jalapeño, and green onions.
4. Divide the oatmeal between two bowls, top each with half of the diced avocado and sprinkle with cilantro.
5. Serve warm and enjoy the blend of savory flavors.

Kcal: 280, Cho: 39g, Fat: 11g, Na: 300mg, Pro: 6g

Banana Pancakes

Servings: 2

Prep Time: 10 minutes

Cook Time: 10 minutes

Ingredients:

- 2 ripe bananas, mashed (200g)
- 2 eggs (100g)
- 1/2 cup whole wheat flour (60g)
- 1/2 teaspoon baking powder (2g)

- 1/4 teaspoon cinnamon (1g)
- 1/2 teaspoon vanilla extract (2ml)
- 1 tablespoon olive oil for cooking (15ml)

Instructions:

1. In a mixing bowl, combine mashed bananas, eggs, whole wheat flour, baking powder, cinnamon, and vanilla extract.
2. Heat olive oil in a non-stick skillet over medium heat.
3. Pour 1/4 cup (60ml) of batter for each pancake into the skillet. Cook until bubbles form on the surface, then flip and cook until golden brown on the other side, about 2 minutes per side.
4. Serve hot with your favorite low-calorie syrup or fresh fruits.

Kcal: 280, Cho: 44g, Fat: 8g, Na: 200mg, Pro: 8g

Tomato Basil Omelet

Servings: 2

Prep Time: 5 minutes

Cook Time: 8 minutes

Ingredients:

- 4 eggs (200g)
- 1/2 cup chopped tomatoes (90g)
- 1/4 cup shredded low-fat mozzarella cheese (30g)
- 2 tablespoons chopped fresh basil (8g)
- Salt and pepper to taste
- 1 teaspoon olive oil (5ml)

Instructions:

1. In a bowl, whisk together eggs, salt, and pepper.
2. Heat olive oil in a non-stick skillet over medium heat. Pour in the egg mixture.
3. As the eggs begin to set, sprinkle chopped tomatoes, basil, and mozzarella over half of the omelet.
4. Fold the other half over the filling and continue cooking until the cheese melts, about 2 minutes.
5. Carefully slide the omelet onto a plate, cut in half, and serve immediately.

Kcal: 215, Cho: 3g, Fat: 15g, Na: 310mg, Pro: 16g

Berry Quinoa Breakfast Bowl

Servings: 2

Prep Time: 5 minutes

Cook Time: 20 minutes

Ingredients:

- 1/2 cup quinoa (85g)
- 1 cup water (240ml)
- 1/2 cup fresh blueberries (75g)
- 1/2 cup sliced strawberries (75g)
- 1/4 cup chopped nuts (almonds or walnuts) (30g)
- 1/4 teaspoon liquid stevia (or to taste)

Instructions:

1. Rinse quinoa under cold water and drain.
2. In a small saucepan, bring quinoa and water to a boil. Reduce heat to low, cover, and simmer until quinoa is tender and water is absorbed, about 15 minutes.
3. Remove from heat and let sit covered for 5 minutes. Fluff with a fork.
4. Divide quinoa into two bowls, and top with blueberries, strawberries, and nuts.
5. Drizzle with liquid stevia to match your sweetness preference, as stevia's sweetness can vary.
6. Serve warm for a nutritious start to your day.

Kcal: 285, Cho: 45g, Fat: 10g, Na: 5mg, Pro: 6g

Almond and Banana Smoothie

Servings: 2

Prep Time: 5 minutes

Cook Time: 0 minutes

Ingredients:

- 2 bananas (200g)
- 1 cup unsweetened almond milk (240ml)
- 1/2 cup Greek yogurt (low-fat) (120g)
- 2 tablespoons almond butter (32g)
- 1/8 teaspoon liquid stevia (or to taste)
- Ice cubes (optional)

Instructions:

1. Place bananas, almond milk, Greek yogurt, almond butter, liquid stevia, and ice cubes (if using) in a blender.
2. Blend on high speed until smooth and creamy.
3. Pour into glasses and serve immediately for a refreshing and filling drink.

Kcal: 315, Cho: 40g, Fat: 14g, Na: 90mg, Pro: 10g

Egg White Scramble with Spinach

Servings: 2

Prep Time: 5 minutes

Cook Time: 5 minutes

Ingredients:

- 1 cup egg whites (240ml)
- 1 cup fresh spinach, chopped (30g)
- 1/2 cup cherry tomatoes, halved (75g)
- 1/4 cup feta cheese, crumbled (50g)
- Salt and pepper to taste
- 1 teaspoon olive oil (5ml)

Instructions:

1. Heat olive oil in a non-stick skillet over medium heat (350°F / 177°C).
2. Add the egg whites and cook, stirring frequently, until they begin to set.
3. Stir in the spinach and cherry tomatoes, cooking until the spinach wilts and the eggs are fully cooked.
4. Season with salt and pepper, then sprinkle with feta cheese.
5. Serve warm for a protein-rich start to your day.

Kcal: 150, Cho: 3g, Fat: 8g, Na: 400mg, Pro: 18g

Peach and Chia Pudding

Servings: 2

Prep Time: 10 minutes (plus chilling)

Cook Time: 0 minutes

Ingredients:

- 2 peaches, pitted and sliced (300g)
- 1/4 cup chia seeds (40g)

- 1 cup almond milk (240ml)
- 1/8 teaspoon liquid stevia (or to taste)
- 1/2 teaspoon vanilla extract (2ml)

Instructions:

1. In a bowl, mix the chia seeds, almond milk, stevia, and vanilla extract.
2. Divide the sliced peaches between two serving glasses.
3. Pour the chia mixture over the peaches evenly.
4. Refrigerate for at least 2 hours or overnight until the pudding sets.
5. Stir before serving to ensure the mixture is evenly distributed.

Kcal: 210, Cho: 31g, Fat: 7g, Na: 30mg, Pro: 5g

Cottage Cheese and Pineapple Plate

Servings: 2

Prep Time: 5 minutes

Cook Time: 0 minutes

Ingredients:

- 1 cup low-fat cottage cheese (225g)
- 1 cup pineapple chunks, fresh or canned in juice (165g)
- 2 tablespoons shredded coconut, unsweetened (15g)

Instructions:

1. Divide the cottage cheese between two plates.
2. Top each serving with pineapple chunks.
3. Sprinkle shredded coconut over the top.
4. Serve immediately as a refreshing and healthy snack or dessert.

Kcal: 200, Cho: 20g, Fat: 5g, Na: 500mg, Pro: 14g

Multigrain Waffles

Servings: 2

Prep Time: 10 minutes

Cook Time: 5 minutes

Ingredients:

- 1 cup multigrain flour (120g)
- 1 cup skim milk (240ml)
- 1 egg (50g)
- 2 tablespoons olive oil (30ml)
- 1 tablespoon sugar (12g)
- 2 teaspoons baking powder (10g)
- 1/4 teaspoon salt (1g)

Instructions:

1. Preheat your waffle iron to medium-high (375°F / 190°C).
2. In a large bowl, whisk together multigrain flour, baking powder, sugar, and salt.
3. In another bowl, beat the egg with milk and olive oil.
4. Combine the wet and dry ingredients until smooth.
5. Pour the batter onto the hot waffle iron and cook until golden and crisp.
6. Serve the waffles hot with your favorite low-fat toppings.

Kcal: 380, Cho: 50g, Fat: 16g, Na: 800mg, Pro: 11g

Southwest Tofu Scramble

Servings: 2

Prep Time: 10 minutes

Cook Time: 10 minutes

Ingredients:

- 1 block firm tofu, drained and crumbled (400g)
- 1/2 cup black beans, rinsed and drained (85g)
- 1/2 red bell pepper, diced (75g)
- 1/2 onion, diced (50g)
- 1 teaspoon cumin (2g)
- 1/2 teaspoon chili powder (1g)
- Salt and pepper to taste
- 1 tablespoon olive oil (15ml)

Instructions:

1. Heat olive oil in a non-stick skillet over medium heat (350°F / 177°C).
2. Add the onion and bell pepper, sautéing until softened.
3. Stir in the crumbled tofu, black beans, cumin, and chili powder.
4. Cook, stirring frequently, for about 5-7 minutes or until the tofu is thoroughly heated and begins to brown.
5. Season with salt and pepper.

6. Serve warm, topped with fresh cilantro or avocado if desired.

Kcal: 320, Cho: 28g, Fat: 18g, Na: 300mg, Pro: 22g

Baked Blueberry Oatmeal Cups

Servings: 2

Prep Time: 10 minutes

Cook Time: 20 minutes

Ingredients:

- 1 cup rolled oats (90g)
- 1/2 cup fresh blueberries (75g)
- 1 banana, mashed (120g)
- 1 cup unsweetened almond milk (240ml)
- 1 teaspoon vanilla extract (5ml)
- 1/16 teaspoon liquid stevia (or to taste)
- 1/2 teaspoon baking powder (2g)

Instructions:

1. Preheat the oven to 375°F (190°C).
2. In a bowl, combine oats, baking powder, mashed banana, almond milk, vanilla extract, and stevia.
3. Gently fold in blueberries.
4. Divide the mixture evenly into a greased muffin tin.
5. Bake for 20 minutes or until the tops are golden and a toothpick inserted into the center comes out clean.
6. Allow to cool before serving.

Kcal: 275, Cho: 50g, Fat: 5g, Na: 80mg, Pro: 6g

Green Tea Smoothie

Servings: 2

Prep Time: 5 minutes

Cook Time: 0 minutes

Ingredients:

- 1 cup brewed green tea, cooled (240ml)
- 1 banana (120g)

- 1/2 cup spinach leaves (15g)
- 1/2 avocado (100g)
- 1/16 teaspoon liquid stevia (or to taste)
- Ice cubes

Instructions:

1. Place all ingredients in a blender, including the liquid stevia.
2. Blend on high until smooth.
3. Serve immediately for a refreshing, antioxidant-rich smoothie.

Kcal: 185, Cho: 28g, Fat: 7g, Na: 20mg, Pro: 2g

Veggie-Packed Breakfast Burrito

Servings: 2

Prep Time: 10 minutes

Cook Time: 10 minutes

Ingredients:

- 4 large eggs (200g)
- 1/2 cup diced bell peppers (75g)
- 1/4 cup diced onions (40g)
- 1/2 cup chopped spinach (15g)
- 2 whole wheat tortillas (90g)
- 1/4 cup shredded low-fat cheese (30g)
- 1 tablespoon olive oil (15ml)
- Salt and pepper to taste

Instructions:

1. Heat olive oil in a skillet over medium heat (350°F / 177°C).
2. Sauté onions and bell peppers until soft.
3. Beat eggs and pour over the vegetables, add spinach, and cook, stirring until the eggs are set.
4. Warm the tortillas, divide the egg mixture between them, sprinkle with cheese.
5. Roll up the tortillas, serve warm.

Kcal: 325, Cho: 28g, Fat: 18g, Na: 320mg, Pro: 19g

Apple Cinnamon Porridge

Servings: 2

Prep Time: 5 minutes

Cook Time: 10 minutes

Ingredients:

- 1 cup rolled oats (90g)
- 2 cups water (480ml)
- 1 apple, peeled and diced (120g)
- 1/2 teaspoon cinnamon (1g)
- 1/16 teaspoon liquid stevia (or to taste)
- 1/4 cup chopped walnuts (30g)

Instructions:

1. Bring water to a boil in a saucepan, add oats, and reduce heat.
2. Simmer for 5 minutes, stirring occasionally.
3. Add diced apple and cinnamon, and continue to cook for another 5 minutes.
4. Stir in stevia and walnuts before serving.

Kcal: 265, Cho: 42g, Fat: 8g, Na: 10mg, Pro: 6g

Pumpkin Spice Latte Smoothie

Servings: 2

Prep Time: 5 minutes

Cook Time: 0 minutes

Ingredients:

- 1/2 cup pumpkin puree (115g)
- 1 banana (120g)
- 1 cup unsweetened almond milk (240ml)
- 1/2 teaspoon pumpkin pie spice (1g)
- 1 tablespoon maple syrup (15g)
- Ice cubes

Instructions:

1. Combine pumpkin puree, banana, almond milk, pumpkin pie spice, maple syrup, and ice in a blender.
2. Blend on high until smooth.
3. Pour into glasses and serve chilled for a festive, nutritious treat.

Kcal: 160, Cho: 35g, Fat: 1.5g, Na: 30mg, Pro: 2g

Chapter 7: Luscious Lunches

Grilled Veggie and Hummus Wraps

Servings: 2

Prep Time: 15 minutes

Cook Time: 10 minutes

Ingredients:

- 1 zucchini, sliced lengthwise (200g)
- 1 yellow squash, sliced lengthwise (200g)
- 1 red bell pepper, seeded and quartered (150g)
- 2 tablespoons olive oil (30ml)
- Salt and pepper to taste
- 1/2 cup hummus (120g)
- 2 whole wheat tortillas (90g)
- 1/2 cup arugula (10g)

Instructions:

1. Preheat grill to medium-high (375°F / 190°C).
2. Brush zucchini, yellow squash, and red bell pepper with olive oil; season with salt and pepper.
3. Grill vegetables until tender and charred, about 5 minutes per side.
4. Spread hummus evenly on each tortilla.
5. Arrange grilled vegetables and arugula on top of the hummus.
6. Roll up the tortillas tightly and cut in half.

Kcal: 380, Cho: 45g, Fat: 18g, Na: 420mg, Pro: 12g

Chicken Salad with Mixed Greens

Servings: 2

Prep Time: 10 minutes

Cook Time: 15 minutes

Ingredients:

- 2 chicken breasts, boneless and skinless (400g)
- 1 tablespoon olive oil (15ml)
- 4 cups mixed greens (120g)
- 1/4 cup sliced almonds (30g)
- 1/4 cup dried cranberries (40g)
- 2 tablespoons balsamic vinaigrette (30ml)

Instructions:

1. Heat olive oil in a skillet over medium heat (350°F / 177°C).
2. Cook chicken breasts until golden and no longer pink in the center, about 7 minutes per side.
3. Let chicken rest for 5 minutes, then slice thinly.
4. Toss mixed greens, sliced almonds, dried cranberries, and chicken in a large bowl.
5. Drizzle with balsamic vinaigrette and toss again to combine.
6. Serve immediately.

Kcal: 380, Cho: 20g, Fat: 15g, Na: 300mg, Pro: 35g

Turkey and Bean Chili

Servings: 2

Prep Time: 10 minutes

Cook Time: 30 minutes

Ingredients:

- 1/2 pound ground turkey (225g)
- 1 can black beans, drained and rinsed (15 oz or 425g)
- 1 can diced tomatoes (14.5 oz or 410g)
- 1 onion, chopped (100g)
- 1 green bell pepper, chopped (150g)
- 2 cloves garlic, minced (6g)
- 1 tablespoon chili powder (8g)
- 1 teaspoon cumin (2g)
- 2 cups chicken broth (480ml)
- Salt and pepper to taste

Instructions:

1. In a large pot, cook ground turkey over medium heat (350°F / 177°C) until browned.
2. Add onion, green bell pepper, and garlic; cook until vegetables are softened, about 5 minutes.
3. Stir in chili powder and cumin; cook for 1 minute.
4. Add black beans, diced tomatoes, and chicken broth. Bring to a boil, then reduce heat and simmer for 20 minutes.
5. Season with salt and pepper. Serve hot.

Kcal: 450, Cho: 54g, Fat: 12g, Na: 700mg, Pro: 35g

Quinoa and Black Bean Salad

Servings: 2

Prep Time: 10 minutes

Cook Time: 20 minutes

Ingredients:

- 1/2 cup quinoa (85g)
- 1 cup water (240ml)
- 1 can black beans, drained and rinsed (15 oz or 425g)
- 1 red bell pepper, diced (150g)
- 1/4 cup chopped fresh cilantro (4g)
- Juice of 1 lime (30ml)
- 2 tablespoons olive oil (30ml)
- Salt and pepper to taste

Instructions:

1. Rinse quinoa under cold water until water runs clear.
2. In a saucepan, bring quinoa and water to a boil. Reduce heat to low, cover, and simmer until quinoa is tender and water is absorbed, about 15 minutes.
3. In a large bowl, combine cooked quinoa, black beans, red bell pepper, and cilantro.
4. In a small bowl, whisk together lime juice, olive oil, salt, and pepper.
5. Pour dressing over quinoa mixture and toss to combine.
6. Serve chilled or at room temperature.

Kcal: 400, Cho: 60g, Fat: 14g, Na: 400mg, Pro: 14g

Stuffed Bell Peppers

Servings: 2

Prep Time: 15 minutes

Cook Time: 30 minutes

Ingredients:

- 2 bell peppers, halved and seeded (300g)
- 1/2 cup cooked brown rice (90g)
- 1/2 cup canned corn, drained (80g)
- 1/4 cup black beans, rinsed and drained (40g)
- 1/4 cup tomato sauce (60ml)
- 1/4 cup shredded low-fat cheese (30g)
- 1/2 onion, diced (50g)

- 1 clove garlic, minced (3g)
- 1 teaspoon olive oil (5ml)
- Salt and pepper to taste

Instructions:

1. Preheat oven to 375°F (190°C).
2. In a skillet, heat olive oil over medium heat. Sauté onion and garlic until translucent.
3. Stir in brown rice, corn, black beans, and tomato sauce. Season with salt and pepper.
4. Spoon the mixture into each bell pepper half. Top with shredded cheese.
5. Place stuffed peppers in a baking dish and cover with foil.
6. Bake in the preheated oven for 25 minutes. Remove foil and bake for an additional 5 minutes or until the cheese is bubbly.
7. Serve warm.

Kcal: 300, Cho: 50g, Fat: 8g, Na: 400mg, Pro: 12g

Broccoli and Cauliflower Soup

Servings: 2

Prep Time: 10 minutes

Cook Time: 20 minutes

Ingredients:

- 2 cups broccoli florets (150g)
- 2 cups cauliflower florets (150g)
- 1 onion, chopped (100g)
- 2 cloves garlic, minced (6g)
- 3 cups vegetable broth (720ml)
- 1/2 cup low-fat milk (120ml)
- Salt and pepper to taste
- 1 tablespoon olive oil (15ml)

Instructions:

1. Heat olive oil in a large pot over medium heat (350°F / 177°C).
2. Sauté onion and garlic until soft, about 5 minutes.
3. Add broccoli and cauliflower, cook for another 5 minutes.
4. Pour in vegetable broth, bring to a boil, then simmer for 10 minutes until vegetables are tender.
5. Puree the soup using an immersion blender until smooth.
6. Stir in low-fat milk, season with salt and pepper, and heat through.
7. Serve warm.

Kcal: 180, Cho: 27g, Fat: 7g, Na: 470mg, Pro: 7g

Avocado Tuna Salad

Servings: 2

Prep Time: 10 minutes

Cook Time: 0 minutes

Ingredients:

- 1 can tuna in water, drained (5 oz or 140g)
- 1 ripe avocado, mashed (200g)
- 1/4 cup diced celery (30g)
- 1/4 cup diced red onion (40g)
- 1 tablespoon lemon juice (15ml)
- Salt and pepper to taste

Instructions:

1. In a medium bowl, combine the drained tuna, mashed avocado, celery, red onion, and lemon juice.
2. Mix thoroughly until all ingredients are well combined.
3. Season with salt and pepper to taste.
4. Serve chilled on a bed of lettuce or with whole-grain crackers.

Kcal: 290, Cho: 15g, Fat: 20g, Na: 380mg, Pro: 17g

Veggie and Lentil Soup

Servings: 2

Prep Time: 10 minutes

Cook Time: 30 minutes

Ingredients:

- 1/2 cup dry lentils (100g)
- 1 carrot, diced (60g)
- 1 stalk celery, diced (40g)
- 1/2 onion, diced (50g)
- 2 cloves garlic, minced (6g)
- 3 cups vegetable broth (720ml)
- 1 teaspoon dried thyme (1g)
- 1 bay leaf

- Salt and pepper to taste
- 1 tablespoon olive oil (15ml)

Instructions:

1. Heat olive oil in a large pot over medium heat (350°F / 177°C).
2. Add onion, carrot, celery, and garlic; sauté until vegetables are softened, about 5 minutes.
3. Stir in lentils, thyme, bay leaf, and vegetable broth.
4. Bring to a boil, then reduce heat and simmer covered for 25 minutes, or until lentils are tender.
5. Remove bay leaf, season with salt and pepper, and serve hot.

Kcal: 255, Cho: 38g, Fat: 7g, Na: 480mg, Pro: 14g

Greek Salad with Chicken

Servings: 2

Prep Time: 15 minutes

Cook Time: 10 minutes

Ingredients:

- 2 chicken breasts, grilled and sliced (400g)
- 1 cucumber, sliced (200g)
- 1 tomato, chopped (150g)
- 1/4 cup sliced red onion (40g)
- 1/4 cup feta cheese, crumbled (50g)
- 1/4 cup Kalamata olives, pitted (30g)
- 2 tablespoons olive oil (30ml)
- 1 tablespoon red wine vinegar (15ml)
- 1/2 teaspoon dried oregano (1g)
- Salt and pepper to taste

Instructions:

1. In a large salad bowl, combine cucumber, tomato, red onion, feta cheese, and olives.
2. In a small bowl, whisk together olive oil, red wine vinegar, oregano, salt, and pepper to make the dressing.
3. Drizzle the dressing over the salad and toss to combine.
4. Top with sliced grilled chicken.
5. Serve immediately.

Kcal: 380, Cho: 12g, Fat: 22g, Na: 620mg, Pro: 35g

Spicy Shrimp Stir Fry

Servings: 2

Prep Time: 10 minutes

Cook Time: 10 minutes

Ingredients:

- 1/2 pound shrimp, peeled and deveined (225g)
- 1 bell pepper, sliced (150g)
- 1/2 onion, sliced (50g)
- 1 cup snap peas (100g)
- 2 cloves garlic, minced (6g)
- 1 tablespoon soy sauce (15ml)
- 1 tablespoon oyster sauce (15ml)
- 1 teaspoon chili sauce (5ml)
- 1 tablespoon olive oil (15ml)

Instructions:

1. Heat olive oil in a large skillet over medium-high heat (375°F / 190°C).
2. Add garlic, bell pepper, onion, and snap peas; stir-fry for 5 minutes until vegetables are just tender.
3. Add shrimp and stir-fry for another 3 minutes or until shrimp are pink and cooked through.
4. Stir in soy sauce, oyster sauce, and chili sauce; cook for 1 minute more to coat everything evenly.
5. Serve hot.

Kcal: 295, Cho: 16g, Fat: 12g, Na: 690mg, Pro: 26g

Cauliflower Rice Burrito Bowl

Servings: 2

Prep Time: 10 minutes

Cook Time: 10 minutes

Ingredients:

- 1 head cauliflower, riced (500g)
- 1/2 cup black beans, drained and rinsed (85g)
- 1/2 cup corn kernels (80g)
- 1 avocado, diced (200g)

- 1/2 cup chopped fresh tomato (90g)
- 1/4 cup chopped red onion (40g)
- Juice of 1 lime (30ml)
- 1/4 cup fresh cilantro, chopped (4g)
- 1 tablespoon olive oil (15ml)
- Salt and pepper to taste

Instructions:

1. Heat olive oil in a skillet over medium heat (350°F / 177°C).
2. Add the riced cauliflower, season with salt and pepper, and sauté until tender, about 5 minutes.
3. Divide the cauliflower rice between two bowls.
4. Top each bowl with black beans, corn, avocado, tomato, and red onion.
5. Sprinkle with lime juice and garnish with cilantro.
6. Serve immediately for a fresh, flavorful meal.

Kcal: 315, Cho: 45g, Fat: 14g, Na: 200mg, Pro: 9g

Butternut Squash Soup

Servings: 2

Prep Time: 10 minutes

Cook Time: 30 minutes

Ingredients:

- 2 cups butternut squash, cubed (300g)
- 1 apple, peeled and diced (150g)
- 1 onion, chopped (100g)
- 3 cups vegetable broth (720ml)
- 1/2 teaspoon ground cinnamon (1g)
- 1/4 teaspoon nutmeg (1g)
- Salt and pepper to taste
- 1 tablespoon olive oil (15ml)

Instructions:

1. Heat olive oil in a large pot over medium heat (350°F / 177°C).
2. Sauté onion until translucent, about 5 minutes.
3. Add butternut squash, apple, cinnamon, nutmeg, and vegetable broth.
4. Bring to a boil, then reduce heat and simmer until squash is tender, about 25 minutes.
5. Puree the soup using an immersion blender until smooth.
6. Season with salt and pepper, and serve warm.

Kcal: 210, Cho: 50g, Fat: 4g, Na: 480mg, Pro: 3g

Spinach and Strawberry Salad

Servings: 2

Prep Time: 10 minutes

Cook Time: 0 minutes

Ingredients:

- 4 cups fresh spinach (120g)
- 1 cup strawberries, sliced (150g)
- 1/4 cup slivered almonds (30g)
- 2 tablespoons balsamic vinaigrette (30ml)
- 1/4 cup crumbled feta cheese (50g)

Instructions:

1. In a large bowl, combine spinach, sliced strawberries, and slivered almonds.
2. Drizzle with balsamic vinaigrette and toss to combine.
3. Sprinkle with crumbled feta cheese.
4. Serve immediately for a refreshing and nutritious salad.

Kcal: 200, Cho: 18g, Fat: 12g, Na: 320mg, Pro: 8g

Zucchini Noodles with Pesto

Servings: 2

Prep Time: 10 minutes

Cook Time: 5 minutes

Ingredients:

- 2 zucchinis, spiralized (400g)
- 1/4 cup basil pesto (60ml)
- 1/4 cup cherry tomatoes, halved (37g)
- 1 tablespoon pine nuts (8g)
- Salt and pepper to taste

Instructions:

1. Heat a non-stick skillet over medium heat (350°F / 177°C).

2. Add spiralized zucchini, salt, and pepper, and sauté for about 2-3 minutes until just tender.
3. Remove from heat and stir in basil pesto.
4. Top with cherry tomatoes and pine nuts.
5. Serve warm as a light, flavorful dish.

Kcal: 255, Cho: 18g, Fat: 18g, Na: 380mg, Pro: 6g

Chicken and Veggie Kabobs

Servings: 2

Prep Time: 15 minutes (plus marinating)

Cook Time: 10 minutes

Ingredients:

- 1/2 pound chicken breast, cut into chunks (225g)
- 1 bell pepper, cut into pieces (150g)
- 1 zucchini, sliced (200g)
- 1 onion, cut into wedges (100g)
- 2 tablespoons olive oil (30ml)
- 1 tablespoon lemon juice (15ml)
- 1 teaspoon dried oregano (1g)
- Salt and pepper to taste

Instructions:

1. In a bowl, mix olive oil, lemon juice, oregano, salt, and pepper.
2. Add chicken and vegetables, toss to coat, and marinate for at least 30 minutes.
3. Preheat the grill to medium-high (375°F / 190°C).
4. Thread chicken and vegetables onto skewers.
5. Grill, turning occasionally, until chicken is cooked through and vegetables are charred, about 10 minutes.
6. Serve hot.

Kcal: 325, Cho: 12g, Fat: 18g, Na: 150mg, Pro: 28g

Turkey Lettuce Wraps

Servings: 2

Prep Time: 10 minutes

Cook Time: 10 minutes

Ingredients:

- 1/2 pound ground turkey (225g)
- 1 carrot, shredded (60g)
- 1/4 cup water chestnuts, diced (30g)
- 1 green onion, chopped (15g)
- 1 clove garlic, minced (3g)
- 1 tablespoon hoisin sauce (15ml)
- 1 tablespoon soy sauce (15ml)
- 1 teaspoon sesame oil (5ml)
- 6 leaves of iceberg lettuce (150g)

Instructions:

1. Heat a skillet over medium heat (350°F / 177°C) and cook the ground turkey until browned.
2. Add garlic, carrot, and water chestnuts, cooking for another 5 minutes until vegetables are soft.
3. Stir in hoisin sauce, soy sauce, and sesame oil, and cook for 2 more minutes.
4. Spoon the turkey mixture into the center of each lettuce leaf.
5. Garnish with green onions and serve immediately.

Kcal: 250, Cho: 15g, Fat: 10g, Na: 620mg, Pro: 28g

Asian Chicken Salad

Servings: 2

Prep Time: 15 minutes

Cook Time: 10 minutes

Ingredients:

- 2 chicken breasts, cooked and shredded (400g)
- 2 cups shredded cabbage (150g)
- 1 carrot, julienned (60g)
- 1/2 red bell pepper, thinly sliced (75g)
- 2 tablespoons chopped cilantro (8g)
- 2 tablespoons sliced almonds (15g)
- 3 tablespoons low-fat Asian dressing (45ml)

Instructions:

1. In a large bowl, combine shredded chicken, cabbage, carrot, red bell pepper, and cilantro.

2. Add Asian dressing and toss to coat evenly.
3. Sprinkle with sliced almonds.
4. Serve chilled, allowing flavors to blend for a refreshing meal.

Kcal: 320, Cho: 18g, Fat: 12g, Na: 410mg, Pro: 35g

Eggplant and Tomato Stew

Servings: 2

Prep Time: 10 minutes

Cook Time: 25 minutes

Ingredients:

- 1 eggplant, cubed (300g)
- 2 tomatoes, chopped (200g)
- 1 onion, chopped (100g)
- 2 cloves garlic, minced (6g)
- 1 tablespoon olive oil (15ml)
- 1/2 teaspoon dried basil (1g)
- Salt and pepper to taste

Instructions:

1. Heat olive oil in a pot over medium heat (350°F / 177°C).
2. Sauté onion and garlic until translucent.
3. Add eggplant and tomatoes, season with basil, salt, and pepper.
4. Cover and simmer for 20 minutes until vegetables are tender and flavors meld.
5. Serve hot, perfect with crusty bread or as a hearty side dish.

Kcal: 180, Cho: 27g, Fat: 7g, Na: 15mg, Pro: 4g

Spiced Lentil Tacos

Servings: 2

Prep Time: 10 minutes

Cook Time: 20 minutes

Ingredients:

- 1 cup cooked lentils (200g)
- 1/2 teaspoon chili powder (1g)
- 1/2 teaspoon cumin (1g)

- 4 corn tortillas (120g)
- 1/2 cup diced tomatoes (75g)
- 1/4 cup diced onion (40g)
- 1/4 cup fresh cilantro, chopped (4g)
- Lime wedges for serving

Instructions:

1. Heat lentils in a skillet over medium heat (350°F / 177°C). Season with chili powder and cumin.
2. Warm tortillas in the same skillet for about 30 seconds on each side.
3. Divide the spiced lentils among the tortillas.
4. Top each taco with tomatoes, onion, and cilantro.
5. Serve with lime wedges on the side.

Kcal: 280, Cho: 42g, Fat: 3g, Na: 30mg, Pro: 14g

Curried Veggie Wrap

Servings: 2

Prep Time: 10 minutes

Cook Time: 10 minutes

Ingredients:

- 1/2 cup cauliflower, chopped (50g)
- 1/2 cup chickpeas, drained and rinsed (85g)
- 1/2 cup spinach leaves (15g)
- 1/2 carrot, julienned (30g)
- 2 whole wheat tortillas (90g)
- 1 tablespoon curry powder (8g)
- 1 tablespoon low-fat Greek yogurt (15ml)
- 1 teaspoon olive oil (5ml)

Instructions:

1. Heat olive oil in a skillet over medium heat (350°F / 177°C). Add cauliflower and chickpeas; sprinkle with curry powder.
2. Cook for 5 minutes, stirring occasionally, until vegetables are tender.
3. Remove from heat and let cool slightly.
4. Spread Greek yogurt on each tortilla.
5. Divide the vegetable mixture between the tortillas, top with spinach and carrot.
6. Roll up tightly and slice in half to serve.

Kcal: 270, Cho: 45g, Fat: 7g, Na: 180mg, Pro: 11g

Chapter 8: Divine Dinners

Herb-Roasted Chicken Breast

Servings: 2

Prep Time: 10 minutes

Cook Time: 25 minutes

Ingredients:

- 2 chicken breasts, boneless and skinless (400g)
- 1 tablespoon olive oil (15ml)
- 1 teaspoon dried rosemary (1g)
- 1 teaspoon dried thyme (1g)
- 1/2 teaspoon garlic powder (1g)
- Salt and pepper to taste

Instructions:

1. Preheat the oven to 375°F (190°C).
2. Rub each chicken breast with olive oil and season with rosemary, thyme, garlic powder, salt, and pepper.
3. Place chicken in a baking dish and roast in the preheated oven until the chicken is cooked through and juices run clear, about 25 minutes.
4. Let rest for 5 minutes before slicing to serve.

Kcal: 230, Cho: 0g, Fat: 10g, Na: 65mg, Pro: 34g

Baked Salmon with Asparagus

Servings: 2

Prep Time: 5 minutes

Cook Time: 20 minutes

Ingredients:

- 2 salmon fillets (6 oz each or 170g each)
- 1 bunch asparagus, trimmed (200g)
- 1 tablespoon olive oil (15ml)
- Lemon slices for garnish
- Salt and pepper to taste

Instructions:

1. Preheat the oven to 400°F (204°C).

2. Arrange the asparagus in a single layer on a baking sheet, drizzle with half the olive oil, and season with salt and pepper.
3. Place the salmon fillets among the asparagus. Drizzle with the remaining olive oil and season with salt and pepper.
4. Bake for 20 minutes, or until salmon is flaky and asparagus is tender.
5. Serve garnished with lemon slices.

Kcal: 300, Cho: 5g, Fat: 18g, Na: 75mg, Pro: 30g

Vegetable Stir Fry with Tofu

Servings: 2

Prep Time: 10 minutes

Cook Time: 10 minutes

Ingredients:

- 1/2 block tofu, pressed and cubed (200g)
- 1 bell pepper, sliced (150g)
- 1 carrot, julienned (60g)
- 1 cup broccoli florets (90g)
- 2 tablespoons soy sauce (30ml)
- 1 tablespoon sesame oil (15ml)
- 1 teaspoon grated ginger (2g)
- 1 clove garlic, minced (3g)

Instructions:

1. Heat sesame oil in a large skillet over medium-high heat (375°F / 190°C).
2. Add tofu and cook until golden on all sides, about 5 minutes.
3. Add bell pepper, carrot, broccoli, ginger, and garlic. Stir-fry for another 5 minutes.
4. Drizzle with soy sauce and toss to coat evenly.
5. Serve hot.

Kcal: 255, Cho: 15g, Fat: 16g, Na: 920mg, Pro: 12g

Turkey Meatballs with Zucchini Noodles

Servings: 2

Prep Time: 15 minutes

Cook Time: 20 minutes

Ingredients:

- 1/2 pound ground turkey (225g)
- 1/4 cup breadcrumbs (30g)
- 1 egg (50g)
- 1/4 cup grated Parmesan cheese (25g)
- 1 tablespoon chopped parsley (4g)
- 1 clove garlic, minced (3g)
- 2 zucchinis, spiralized (400g)
- 1 tablespoon olive oil (15ml)
- Salt and pepper to taste

Instructions:

1. Preheat the oven to 375°F (190°C).
2. In a bowl, mix together ground turkey, breadcrumbs, egg, Parmesan, parsley, garlic, salt, and pepper.
3. Form into small meatballs and place on a baking sheet.
4. Bake for 20 minutes or until cooked through.
5. Meanwhile, heat olive oil in a skillet over medium heat. Sauté the spiralized zucchini until tender, about 3-5 minutes.
6. Serve meatballs over zucchini noodles.

Kcal: 350, Cho: 20g, Fat: 18g, Na: 450mg, Pro: 28g

Grilled Eggplant with Tomato Salad

Servings: 2

Prep Time: 10 minutes

Cook Time: 10 minutes

Ingredients:

- 1 large eggplant, sliced into 1/2-inch rounds (300g)
- 2 tomatoes, diced (300g)
- 1/4 cup chopped fresh basil (4g)
- 2 tablespoons balsamic vinegar (30ml)
- 1 tablespoon olive oil (15ml)
- Salt and pepper to taste

Instructions:

1. Preheat grill to medium-high (375°F / 190°C).
2. Brush eggplant slices with olive oil and season with salt and pepper.
3. Grill eggplant until tender and grill marks appear, about 5 minutes per side.
4. Combine tomatoes, basil, and balsamic vinegar in a bowl.

5. Serve grilled eggplant topped with tomato salad.

Kcal: 180, Cho: 23g, Fat: 10g, Na: 10mg, Pro: 3g

Pork Tenderloin with Roasted Apples

Servings: 2

Prep Time: 10 minutes

Cook Time: 25 minutes

Ingredients:

- 1 pork tenderloin (12 oz or 340g)
- 2 apples, cored and sliced (300g)
- 1 tablespoon olive oil (15ml)
- 1 teaspoon dried thyme (1g)
- Salt and pepper to taste

Instructions:

1. Preheat the oven to 375°F (190°C).
2. Rub the pork tenderloin with salt, pepper, and thyme.
3. Heat olive oil in an oven-safe skillet over medium-high heat (375°F / 190°C).
4. Brown the pork on all sides, about 5 minutes.
5. Add sliced apples around the pork in the skillet.
6. Transfer the skillet to the oven and roast for 20 minutes, or until the pork reaches an internal temperature of 145°F (63°C).
7. Let rest before slicing and serve with the roasted apples.

Kcal: 295, Cho: 20g, Fat: 12g, Na: 65mg, Pro: 30g

Spaghetti Squash with Marinara Sauce

Servings: 2

Prep Time: 10 minutes

Cook Time: 45 minutes

Ingredients:

- 1 spaghetti squash (2 lb or 900g)
- 1 cup marinara sauce (240ml)
- 1 tablespoon olive oil (15ml)
- Salt and pepper to taste

- 2 tablespoons grated Parmesan cheese (15g)

Instructions:

1. Preheat the oven to 400°F (204°C).
2. Halve the spaghetti squash lengthwise and remove seeds.
3. Brush the cut sides with olive oil and season with salt and pepper.
4. Place cut side down on a baking sheet and roast until tender, about 40 minutes.
5. Use a fork to shred the squash into strands.
6. Heat marinara sauce in a pan, spoon over the spaghetti squash, and top with Parmesan.
7. Serve hot.

Kcal: 230, Cho: 30g, Fat: 10g, Na: 480mg, Pro: 6g

Veggie-Packed Paella

Servings: 2

Prep Time: 15 minutes

Cook Time: 40 minutes

Ingredients:

- 1/2 cup short-grain rice (90g)
- 1 onion, chopped (100g)
- 1 red bell pepper, chopped (150g)
- 1 tomato, chopped (100g)
- 1/2 cup green peas (75g)
- 1 clove garlic, minced (3g)
- 1/4 teaspoon saffron threads (0.25g)
- 2 cups vegetable broth (480ml)
- 2 tablespoons olive oil (30ml)
- Salt and pepper to taste

Instructions:

1. Heat olive oil in a large skillet over medium heat (350°F / 177°C).
2. Add onion, bell pepper, and garlic. Sauté until softened, about 5 minutes.
3. Stir in rice, chopped tomato, saffron, and vegetable broth.
4. Bring to a boil, then reduce heat to low and simmer covered for 30 minutes.
5. Add green peas and cook uncovered for an additional 10 minutes.
6. Season with salt and pepper and serve hot.

Kcal: 360, Cho: 65g, Fat: 10g, Na: 600mg, Pro: 8g

Moroccan Vegetable Tagine

Servings: 2

Prep Time: 10 minutes

Cook Time: 30 minutes

Ingredients:

- 1 carrot, sliced (60g)
- 1 zucchini, sliced (150g)
- 1/2 cup chickpeas, drained and rinsed (85g)
- 1/2 onion, chopped (50g)
- 2 tomatoes, chopped (200g)
- 1 teaspoon ground cumin (2g)
- 1/2 teaspoon ground cinnamon (1g)
- 1/4 teaspoon ground ginger (0.5g)
- 2 cups vegetable broth (480ml)
- 2 tablespoons olive oil (30ml)
- Salt and pepper to taste

Instructions:

1. Heat olive oil in a large pot over medium heat (350°F / 177°C).
2. Add onions and sauté until translucent.
3. Add carrots, zucchini, spices, and stir to coat.
4. Pour in vegetable broth and bring to a simmer.
5. Add tomatoes and chickpeas, cover, and cook for 20 minutes until vegetables are tender.
6. Season with salt and pepper, and serve hot with couscous.

Kcal: 290, Cho: 40g, Fat: 14g, Na: 480mg, Pro: 8g

Balsamic Glazed Beef

Servings: 2

Prep Time: 5 minutes

Cook Time: 15 minutes

Ingredients:

- 1/2 pound beef tenderloin (225g)
- 2 tablespoons balsamic vinegar (30ml)
- 1/16 teaspoon powdered stevia (or to taste)
- 1 clove garlic, minced (3g)

- 1 tablespoon olive oil (15ml)
- Salt and pepper to taste

Instructions:

1. Heat olive oil in a skillet over medium-high heat (375°F / 190°C).
2. Season the beef with salt and pepper and sear until browned on all sides, about 5 minutes.
3. Lower the heat to medium, add minced garlic, and cook for 1 minute.
4. Mix balsamic vinegar and stevia, pour over the beef, and cook for an additional 5 minutes, basting with the glaze frequently.
5. Slice the beef and serve drizzled with the remaining glaze.

Kcal: 340, Cho: 12g, Fat: 20g, Na: 85mg, Pro: 25g

Lemon Garlic Shrimp Skewers

Servings: 2

Prep Time: 10 minutes

Cook Time: 5 minutes

Ingredients:

- 12 large shrimp, peeled and deveined (340g)
- 2 cloves garlic, minced (6g)
- Juice of 1 lemon (30ml)
- 1 tablespoon olive oil (15ml)
- Salt and pepper to taste
- 4 wooden skewers, soaked in water

Instructions:

1. In a bowl, combine garlic, lemon juice, olive oil, salt, and pepper.
2. Add shrimp and marinate for 10 minutes.
3. Preheat grill to medium-high (375°F / 190°C).
4. Thread shrimp onto skewers.
5. Grill shrimp for 2-3 minutes per side or until opaque and slightly charred.
6. Serve immediately.

Kcal: 195, Cho: 3g, Fat: 8g, Na: 210mg, Pro: 28g

Cauliflower Steak with Olive Relish

Servings: 2

Prep Time: 10 minutes

Cook Time: 20 minutes

Ingredients:

- 1 large head cauliflower (600g)
- 2 tablespoons olive oil (30ml)
- 1/4 cup chopped olives (30g)
- 2 tablespoons chopped parsley (8g)
- 1 tablespoon capers, rinsed and chopped (8g)
- 1 teaspoon lemon zest (2g)
- Salt and pepper to taste

Instructions:

1. Preheat oven to 400°F (204°C).
2. Cut two 1-inch thick slices from the center of the cauliflower to form steaks.
3. Brush both sides with olive oil and season with salt and pepper.
4. Roast in the oven for 20 minutes, flipping halfway through.
5. Mix olives, parsley, capers, and lemon zest to make the relish.
6. Top cauliflower steaks with olive relish and serve.

Kcal: 180, Cho: 11g, Fat: 14g, Na: 380mg, Pro: 5g

Grilled Tilapia with Mango Salsa

Servings: 2

Prep Time: 15 minutes

Cook Time: 10 minutes

Ingredients:

- 2 tilapia fillets (340g)
- 1 mango, peeled and diced (150g)
- 1/4 cup diced red bell pepper (37g)
- 1/4 cup diced red onion (40g)
- 1 tablespoon chopped cilantro (4g)
- Juice of 1 lime (30ml)
- 1 tablespoon olive oil (15ml)
- Salt and pepper to taste

Instructions:

1. Preheat grill to medium (350°F / 177°C).

2. Brush tilapia with olive oil, season with salt and pepper.
3. Grill tilapia for about 5 minutes per side or until fish flakes easily with a fork.
4. Mix mango, bell pepper, onion, cilantro, and lime juice to make the salsa.
5. Serve tilapia topped with mango salsa.

Kcal: 285, Cho: 20g, Fat: 9g, Na: 75mg, Pro: 35g

Beef and Broccoli Stir Fry

Servings: 2

Prep Time: 10 minutes

Cook Time: 10 minutes

Ingredients:

- 1/2 pound beef sirloin, thinly sliced (225g)
- 2 cups broccoli florets (180g)
- 1 tablespoon soy sauce (15ml)
- 1 tablespoon oyster sauce (15ml)
- 1 clove garlic, minced (3g)
- 1 teaspoon grated ginger (2g)
- 1 tablespoon vegetable oil (15ml)

Instructions:

1. Heat oil in a skillet over high heat (400°F / 204°C).
2. Add beef and stir-fry for 2 minutes.
3. Add broccoli, garlic, and ginger, cook for another 5 minutes.
4. Stir in soy sauce and oyster sauce, cook until sauce thickens.
5. Serve immediately.

Kcal: 275, Cho: 10g, Fat: 15g, Na: 600mg, Pro: 25g

Ratatouille

Servings: 2

Prep Time: 15 minutes

Cook Time: 40 minutes

Ingredients:

- 1 small eggplant, cubed (200g)
- 1 zucchini, sliced (150g)

- 1 yellow squash, sliced (150g)
- 1 bell pepper, chopped (150g)
- 1 onion, sliced (100g)
- 2 tomatoes, chopped (200g)
- 3 cloves garlic, minced (9g)
- 2 tablespoons olive oil (30ml)
- 1 teaspoon dried thyme (1g)
- Salt and pepper to taste

Instructions:

1. Preheat the oven to 375°F (190°C).
2. Heat olive oil in a large oven-safe skillet over medium heat (350°F / 177°C).
3. Sauté onion and garlic until softened, about 5 minutes.
4. Add eggplant, zucchini, yellow squash, and bell pepper. Cook for 10 minutes, stirring occasionally.
5. Stir in tomatoes, thyme, salt, and pepper.
6. Transfer skillet to the oven and bake for 25 minutes, or until vegetables are tender and flavors have melded.
7. Serve hot as a side dish or over rice.

Kcal: 220, Cho: 30g, Fat: 12g, Na: 20mg, Pro: 5g

Roast Turkey with Cranberry Sauce

Servings: 2

Prep Time: 10 minutes

Cook Time: 30 minutes

Ingredients:

- 2 turkey breast cutlets (10 oz or 280g)
- 1 tablespoon olive oil (15ml)
- 1 teaspoon dried thyme (1g)
- Salt and pepper to taste
- 1 cup fresh cranberries (100g)
- 1/4 cup orange juice (60ml)
- 1/16 teaspoon liquid stevia (or to taste)

Instructions:

1. Preheat the oven to 375°F (190°C).
2. Rub turkey breast cutlets with olive oil, thyme, salt, and pepper.

3. Place turkey on a baking sheet and roast for 25-30 minutes, or until the internal temperature reaches 165°F (74°C).
4. In a small saucepan, combine cranberries, orange juice, and stevia. Cook over medium heat until cranberries burst and the sauce thickens, about 10 minutes. Adjust the amount of stevia based on your taste preference.
5. Serve the turkey with cranberry sauce on top.

Kcal: 310, Cho: 17g, Fat: 10g, Na: 70mg, Pro: 40g

Coconut Curry with Chickpeas

Servings: 2

Prep Time: 10 minutes

Cook Time: 20 minutes

Ingredients:

- 1 can chickpeas, drained and rinsed (15 oz or 425g)
- 1 cup light coconut milk (240ml)
- 1 onion, chopped (100g)
- 2 cloves garlic, minced (6g)
- 1 tablespoon curry powder (8g)
- 1/2 teaspoon ground cumin (1g)
- 1 tablespoon olive oil (15ml)
- Salt and pepper to taste
- 1/4 cup chopped fresh cilantro (4g)

Instructions:

1. Heat olive oil in a large skillet over medium heat (350°F / 177°C).
2. Sauté onion and garlic until softened, about 5 minutes.
3. Add curry powder and cumin, stirring to coat the onions.
4. Pour in coconut milk and add chickpeas. Simmer for 10 minutes until the sauce thickens.
5. Season with salt and pepper, and stir in fresh cilantro before serving.

Kcal: 280, Cho: 30g, Fat: 14g, Na: 400mg, Pro: 8g

Grilled Portobello Mushrooms

Servings: 2

Prep Time: 5 minutes

Cook Time: 10 minutes

Ingredients:

- 4 large Portobello mushrooms (400g)
- 2 tablespoons balsamic vinegar (30ml)
- 1 tablespoon olive oil (15ml)
- 2 cloves garlic, minced (6g)
- Salt and pepper to taste

Instructions:

1. Preheat grill to medium-high (375°F / 190°C).
2. In a bowl, mix balsamic vinegar, olive oil, garlic, salt, and pepper.
3. Brush the mushrooms with the marinade on both sides.
4. Grill mushrooms for about 5 minutes per side, until tender and slightly charred.
5. Serve hot as a side dish or a meat substitute.

Kcal: 180, Cho: 12g, Fat: 14g, Na: 10mg, Pro: 4g

Stuffed Acorn Squash

Servings: 2

Prep Time: 10 minutes

Cook Time: 40 minutes

Ingredients:

- 1 acorn squash, halved and seeded (600g)
- 1/2 cup quinoa, cooked (90g)
- 1/4 cup dried cranberries (30g)
- 1/4 cup chopped walnuts (30g)
- 1 tablespoon maple syrup (15ml)
- 1 teaspoon ground cinnamon (1g)
- Salt and pepper to taste

Instructions:

1. Preheat the oven to 375°F (190°C).
2. Place acorn squash halves cut side down on a baking sheet. Roast for 30 minutes, until tender.
3. In a bowl, mix cooked quinoa, cranberries, walnuts, maple syrup, cinnamon, salt, and pepper.
4. Remove squash from the oven and fill each half with the quinoa mixture.

5. Return to the oven for 10 minutes to heat through.
6. Serve hot.

Kcal: 300, Cho: 50g, Fat: 10g, Na: 20mg, Pro: 6g

Slow Cooker Pulled Chicken

Servings: 2

Prep Time: 10 minutes

Cook Time: 4 hours

Ingredients:

- 2 chicken breasts (12 oz or 340g)
- 1 cup low-sodium chicken broth (240ml)
- 1/2 cup barbecue sauce (120ml)
- 1 onion, sliced (100g)
- 2 cloves garlic, minced (6g)
- 1 tablespoon olive oil (15ml)
- Salt and pepper to taste

Instructions:

1. Heat olive oil in a skillet over medium heat (350°F / 177°C). Sauté onion and garlic until softened, about 5 minutes.
2. Place chicken breasts in the slow cooker. Add sautéed onions and garlic, chicken broth, and barbecue sauce.
3. Cook on low for 4 hours, or until chicken is tender and easily shredded.
4. Shred the chicken with two forks and mix with the sauce.
5. Serve hot on whole-grain buns or over a salad.

Kcal: 280, Cho: 20g, Fat: 8g, Na: 600mg, Pro: 30g

Chapter 9: Pick-Me-Ups

Carrot and Hummus Dip

Servings: 2

Prep Time: 10 minutes

Cook Time: 0 minutes

Ingredients:

- 4 large carrots, peeled and cut into sticks (240g)
- 1/2 cup hummus (120g)
- 1 tablespoon lemon juice (15ml)
- 1/2 teaspoon ground cumin (1g)
- Salt and pepper to taste

Instructions:

1. In a bowl, mix hummus, lemon juice, cumin, salt, and pepper.
2. Arrange carrot sticks on a plate around the hummus dip.
3. Serve immediately as a healthy snack.

Kcal: 150, Cho: 20g, Fat: 6g, Na: 200mg, Pro: 4g

Greek Yogurt and Mixed Berries

Servings: 2

Prep Time: 5 minutes

Cook Time: 0 minutes

Ingredients:

- 1 cup Greek yogurt (low-fat) (245g)
- 1/2 cup blueberries (75g)
- 1/2 cup strawberries, sliced (75g)
- 1/16 teaspoon liquid stevia (or to taste)
- 1 tablespoon chia seeds (12g)

Instructions:

1. Divide the Greek yogurt between two bowls.
2. Top each serving with blueberries and strawberries.
3. Drizzle liquid stevia over the top, adjusting the amount based on your desired sweetness.
4. Sprinkle chia seeds on top.

5. Serve immediately for a refreshing and nutritious snack.

Kcal: 170, Cho: 22g, Fat: 3g, Na: 50mg, Pro: 10g

Peanut Butter Banana Smoothie

Servings: 2

Prep Time: 5 minutes

Cook Time: 0 minutes

Ingredients:

- 2 bananas (240g)
- 1 cup unsweetened almond milk (240ml)
- 2 tablespoons peanut butter (32g)
- 1/8 teaspoon liquid stevia (or to taste)
- 1/2 cup ice cubes

Instructions:

1. Place bananas, almond milk, peanut butter, stevia, and ice cubes in a blender.
2. Blend on high speed until smooth and creamy.
3. Pour into glasses and serve immediately.

Kcal: 240, Cho: 35g, Fat: 8g, Na: 130mg, Pro: 5g

Spiced Pumpkin Seeds

Servings: 2

Prep Time: 5 minutes

Cook Time: 20 minutes

Ingredients:

- 1 cup raw pumpkin seeds (pepitas) (130g)
- 1 tablespoon olive oil (15ml)
- 1 teaspoon paprika (2g)
- 1/2 teaspoon cayenne pepper (1g)
- 1/2 teaspoon salt (3g)

Instructions:

1. Preheat the oven to 350°F (175°C).

2. In a bowl, mix pumpkin seeds, olive oil, paprika, cayenne pepper, and salt.
3. Spread the seeds in a single layer on a baking sheet.
4. Bake for 20 minutes, stirring halfway through, until golden and crispy.
5. Let cool before serving.

Kcal: 180, Cho: 6g, Fat: 14g, Na: 290mg, Pro: 9g

Cucumber Tomato Salad

Servings: 2

Prep Time: 10 minutes

Cook Time: 0 minutes

Ingredients:

- 1 cucumber, diced (200g)
- 1 cup cherry tomatoes, halved (150g)
- 1/4 red onion, thinly sliced (40g)
- 2 tablespoons olive oil (30ml)
- 1 tablespoon red wine vinegar (15ml)
- Salt and pepper to taste
- 1 tablespoon chopped fresh dill (4g)

Instructions:

1. In a large bowl, combine cucumber, cherry tomatoes, and red onion.
2. Drizzle with olive oil and red wine vinegar, and toss to coat.
3. Season with salt and pepper, and sprinkle with fresh dill.
4. Serve immediately as a light and refreshing side dish.

Kcal: 120, Cho: 10g, Fat: 9g, Na: 10mg, Pro: 2g

Almond Butter Apple Slices

Servings: 2

Prep Time: 5 minutes

Cook Time: 0 minutes

Ingredients:

- 2 apples, cored and sliced (360g)
- 2 tablespoons almond butter (32g)
- 1/16 teaspoon liquid stevia (or to taste)

- 1/4 teaspoon ground cinnamon (1g)

Instructions:

1. Arrange apple slices on a plate.
2. Drizzle almond butter over the apple slices.
3. Drizzle with liquid stevia, adjusting the amount based on your desired sweetness, and sprinkle with cinnamon.
4. Serve immediately as a delicious and nutritious snack.

Kcal: 190, Cho: 35g, Fat: 8g, Na: 5mg, Pro: 2g

Green Detox Smoothie

Servings: 2

Prep Time: 5 minutes

Cook Time: 0 minutes

Ingredients:

- 1 cup spinach leaves (30g)
- 1 cucumber, chopped (200g)
- 1 green apple, cored and chopped (180g)
- 1/2 avocado (100g)
- 1 cup coconut water (240ml)
- Juice of 1 lemon (30ml)

Instructions:

1. Place spinach, cucumber, green apple, avocado, coconut water, and lemon juice in a blender.
2. Blend on high speed until smooth.
3. Pour into glasses and serve immediately for a refreshing detox drink.

Kcal: 160, Cho: 26g, Fat: 8g, Na: 80mg, Pro: 3g

Roasted Chickpeas

Servings: 2

Prep Time: 5 minutes

Cook Time: 30 minutes

Ingredients:

- 1 can chickpeas, drained and rinsed (15 oz or 425g)
- 1 tablespoon olive oil (15ml)
- 1 teaspoon paprika (2g)
- 1/2 teaspoon garlic powder (1g)
- 1/2 teaspoon salt (3g)

Instructions:

1. Preheat the oven to 400°F (204°C).
2. Pat the chickpeas dry with a paper towel and place them in a bowl.
3. Toss with olive oil, paprika, garlic powder, and salt.
4. Spread the chickpeas on a baking sheet in a single layer.
5. Roast for 30 minutes, stirring halfway through, until crispy.
6. Let cool before serving.

Kcal: 190, Cho: 30g, Fat: 7g, Na: 300mg, Pro: 6g

Kale Chips

Servings: 2

Prep Time: 5 minutes

Cook Time: 15 minutes

Ingredients:

- 1 bunch kale, stems removed and torn into pieces (150g)
- 1 tablespoon olive oil (15ml)
- 1/2 teaspoon salt (3g)

Instructions:

1. Preheat the oven to 350°F (175°C).
2. Wash and thoroughly dry the kale pieces.
3. Toss kale with olive oil and salt in a large bowl.
4. Spread in a single layer on a baking sheet.
5. Bake for 15 minutes, or until the edges are brown and crispy.
6. Serve immediately.

Kcal: 100, Cho: 8g, Fat: 7g, Na: 320mg, Pro: 3g

Berry and Spinach Smoothie

Servings: 2

Prep Time: 5 minutes

Cook Time: 0 minutes

Ingredients:

- 1 cup mixed berries (150g)
- 1 cup spinach leaves (30g)
- 1 banana (120g)
- 1 cup almond milk (240ml)
- 1 tablespoon chia seeds (12g)

Instructions:

1. Place mixed berries, spinach, banana, almond milk, and chia seeds in a blender.
2. Blend on high speed until smooth.
3. Pour into glasses and serve immediately for a nutrient-packed smoothie.

Kcal: 180, Cho: 35g, Fat: 5g, Na: 50mg, Pro: 4g

Avocado Egg Salad

Servings: 2

Prep Time: 10 minutes

Cook Time: 10 minutes

Ingredients:

- 4 hard-boiled eggs, chopped (200g)
- 1 avocado, mashed (200g)
- 1 tablespoon Greek yogurt (15g)
- 1 teaspoon Dijon mustard (5g)
- 1 tablespoon lemon juice (15ml)
- Salt and pepper to taste

Instructions:

1. In a medium bowl, combine chopped eggs, mashed avocado, Greek yogurt, Dijon mustard, and lemon juice.
2. Mix until well combined and season with salt and pepper.
3. Serve immediately on whole-grain bread or with lettuce wraps.

Kcal: 210, Cho: 6g, Fat: 16g, Na: 220mg, Pro: 12g

Coconut Yogurt Parfait

Servings: 2

Prep Time: 5 minutes

Cook Time: 0 minutes

Ingredients:

- 1 cup coconut yogurt (245g)
- 1/2 cup granola (60g)
- 1/2 cup mixed berries (75g)
- 1/16 teaspoon liquid stevia (or to taste)
- 1 tablespoon shredded coconut (8g)

Instructions:

1. Divide the coconut yogurt between two bowls or glasses.
2. Layer with granola, mixed berries, and a drizzle of liquid stevia. Adjust the amount of stevia according to your desired sweetness.
3. Sprinkle shredded coconut on top.
4. Serve immediately for a refreshing and healthy snack.

Kcal: 260, Cho: 33g, Fat: 10g, Na: 60mg, Pro: 4g

Air-Popped Popcorn with Sea Salt

Servings: 2

Prep Time: 2 minutes

Cook Time: 5 minutes

Ingredients:

- 1/4 cup popcorn kernels (40g)
- 1/2 teaspoon sea salt (3g)

Instructions:

1. Place popcorn kernels in an air popper and pop according to the manufacturer's instructions.
2. Transfer the popped popcorn to a large bowl.
3. Sprinkle with sea salt and toss to coat evenly.
4. Serve immediately as a light and crunchy snack.

Kcal: 110, Cho: 24g, Fat: 1g, Na: 150mg, Pro: 3g

Beet and Carrot Juice

Servings: 2

Prep Time: 10 minutes

Cook Time: 0 minutes

Ingredients:

- 2 medium beets, peeled and chopped (300g)
- 4 large carrots, peeled and chopped (240g)
- 2 apples, cored and chopped (360g)
- 1-inch piece of ginger, peeled (5g)
- 1 cup water (240ml)

Instructions:

1. Combine beets, carrots, apples, ginger, and water in a blender.
2. Blend on high speed until smooth.
3. Strain the juice through a fine mesh sieve into a pitcher.
4. Serve immediately over ice.

Kcal: 150, Cho: 35g, Fat: 0g, Na: 80mg, Pro: 2g

Watermelon Mint Salad

Servings: 2

Prep Time: 10 minutes

Cook Time: 0 minutes

Ingredients:

- 4 cups watermelon, cubed (600g)
- 1/4 cup fresh mint leaves, chopped (10g)
- 1 tablespoon lime juice (15ml)
- 1/32 teaspoon liquid stevia (or to taste)

Instructions:

1. In a large bowl, combine watermelon cubes and chopped mint leaves.
2. Drizzle with lime juice and liquid stevia, adjusting the amount based on your desired sweetness.
3. Toss gently to combine.
4. Serve immediately as a refreshing and hydrating salad.

Kcal: 85, Cho: 22g, Fat: 0g, Na: 0mg, Pro: 1g

Edamame with Sea Salt

Servings: 2

Prep Time: 5 minutes

Cook Time: 5 minutes

Ingredients:

- 2 cups edamame in pods (300g)
- 1/2 teaspoon sea salt (3g)

Instructions:

1. Bring a pot of water to a boil over medium-high heat (375°F / 190°C).
2. Add the edamame pods and cook for 5 minutes until tender.
3. Drain the edamame and sprinkle with sea salt.
4. Serve warm as a healthy and protein-rich snack.

Kcal: 160, Cho: 13g, Fat: 7g, Na: 250mg, Pro: 12g

Pomegranate Blueberry Blast Smoothie

Servings: 2

Prep Time: 5 minutes

Cook Time: 0 minutes

Ingredients:

- 1 cup pomegranate juice (240ml)
- 1/2 cup blueberries (75g)
- 1 banana (120g)
- 1/2 cup Greek yogurt (120g)
- 1/16 teaspoon liquid stevia (or to taste)

Instructions:

1. Combine pomegranate juice, blueberries, banana, Greek yogurt, and liquid stevia in a blender.
2. Blend on high speed until smooth.
3. Pour into glasses and serve immediately for a refreshing and antioxidant-rich drink.

Kcal: 170, Cho: 35g, Fat: 2g, Na: 40mg, Pro: 5g

Caprese Salad Skewers

Servings: 2

Prep Time: 10 minutes

Cook Time: 0 minutes

Ingredients:

- 12 cherry tomatoes (180g)
- 12 fresh mozzarella balls (120g)
- 12 fresh basil leaves (6g)
- 1 tablespoon balsamic glaze (15ml)
- 1 tablespoon olive oil (15ml)
- Salt and pepper to taste

Instructions:

1. Thread a cherry tomato, mozzarella ball, and basil leaf onto each skewer.
2. Arrange the skewers on a serving plate.
3. Drizzle with olive oil and balsamic glaze.
4. Season with salt and pepper.
5. Serve immediately as a fresh and delightful appetizer.

Kcal: 180, Cho: 7g, Fat: 12g, Na: 200mg, Pro: 8g

Celery and Almond Butter

Servings: 2

Prep Time: 5 minutes

Cook Time: 0 minutes

Ingredients:

- 4 celery stalks, cut into sticks (200g)
- 2 tablespoons almond butter (32g)

Instructions:

1. Arrange the celery sticks on a plate.
2. Serve with almond butter for dipping.
3. Enjoy as a crunchy and nutritious snack.

Kcal: 150, Cho: 10g, Fat: 11g, Na: 75mg, Pro: 4g

Mango Lime Smoothie

Servings: 2

Prep Time: 5 minutes

Cook Time: 0 minutes

Ingredients:

- 1 cup diced mango (165g)
- 1 banana (120g)
- 1 cup coconut water (240ml)
- Juice of 1 lime (30ml)
- 1 tablespoon chia seeds (12g)

Instructions:

1. Combine mango, banana, coconut water, lime juice, and chia seeds in a blender.
2. Blend on high speed until smooth.
3. Pour into glasses and serve immediately for a tropical and refreshing drink.

Kcal: 180, Cho: 40g, Fat: 3g, Na: 30mg, Pro: 3g

Chapter 10: Decadent Desserts

Mixed Berry Sorbet

Servings: 2

Prep Time: 10 minutes

Cook Time: 0 minutes

Ingredients:

- 2 cups mixed berries, frozen (300g)
- 1/4 cup water (60ml)
- 1/8 teaspoon liquid stevia (or to taste)
- 1 tablespoon lemon juice (15ml)

Instructions:

1. Combine mixed berries, water, stevia, and lemon juice in a blender.
2. Blend on high speed until smooth.
3. Transfer the mixture to a freezer-safe container and freeze for at least 2 hours.
4. Scoop into bowls and serve immediately for a refreshing, low-fat treat.

Kcal: 100, Cho: 23g, Fat: 0g, Na: 5mg, Pro: 1g

Baked Apples with Cinnamon

Servings: 2

Prep Time: 10 minutes

Cook Time: 25 minutes

Ingredients:

- 2 large apples, cored and halved (300g)
- 1/16 teaspoon liquid stevia (or to taste)
- 1 teaspoon ground cinnamon (2g)
- 1/4 cup water (60ml)

Instructions:

1. Preheat the oven to 375°F (190°C).
2. Place apple halves in a baking dish and drizzle with liquid stevia, adjusting the amount based on your desired sweetness.
3. Sprinkle with cinnamon and pour water into the dish.
4. Bake for 25 minutes, or until apples are tender.
5. Serve warm as a cozy, guilt-free dessert.

Kcal: 105, Cho: 28g, Fat: 0g, Na: 0mg, Pro: 0g

Strawberry Cheesecake Cups

Servings: 2

Prep Time: 15 minutes

Cook Time: 0 minutes

Ingredients:

- 1 cup Greek yogurt (low-fat) (245g)
- 1/2 cup strawberries, chopped (75g)
- 1/8 teaspoon liquid stevia (or to taste)
- 1/4 teaspoon vanilla extract (1ml)
- 2 graham crackers, crushed (30g)

Instructions:

1. In a bowl, mix Greek yogurt, stevia, and vanilla extract until smooth. Adjust the amount of stevia based on your desired sweetness.
2. Layer the mixture in two cups with chopped strawberries and crushed graham crackers.
3. Refrigerate for 1 hour to set.
4. Serve chilled for a delightful and healthy treat.

Kcal: 165, Cho: 27g, Fat: 2g, Na: 85mg, Pro: 10g

Chocolate Avocado Mousse

Servings: 2

Prep Time: 10 minutes

Cook Time: 0 minutes

Ingredients:

- 1 ripe avocado (200g)
- 2 tablespoons cocoa powder (10g)
- 1/8 teaspoon liquid stevia (or to taste)
- 1/4 cup almond milk (60ml)
- 1 teaspoon vanilla extract (5ml)

Instructions:

1. Scoop the avocado flesh into a blender.
2. Add cocoa powder, stevia, almond milk, and vanilla extract.

3. Blend on high speed until smooth and creamy. Adjust the amount of stevia based on your desired sweetness.
4. Chill in the refrigerator for 1 hour before serving.
5. Serve chilled for a rich and healthy dessert.

Kcal: 210, Cho: 26g, Fat: 10g, Na: 20mg, Pro: 2g

Peach Frozen Yogurt

Servings: 2

Prep Time: 10 minutes

Cook Time: 0 minutes

Ingredients:

- 2 cups peaches, frozen and sliced (300g)
- 1 cup Greek yogurt (low-fat) (245g)
- 1/8 teaspoon liquid stevia (or to taste)
- 1 teaspoon lemon juice (5ml)

Instructions:

1. Combine frozen peaches, Greek yogurt, stevia, and lemon juice in a blender.
2. Blend on high speed until smooth and creamy. Adjust the amount of stevia based on your desired sweetness.
3. Transfer the mixture to a freezer-safe container and freeze for 1 hour.
4. Scoop into bowls and serve immediately for a cool, low-fat dessert.

Kcal: 115, Cho: 22g, Fat: 1g, Na: 30mg, Pro: 5g

Pineapple Carpaccio

Servings: 2

Prep Time: 10 minutes

Cook Time: 0 minutes

Ingredients:

- 1 small pineapple, thinly sliced (300g)
- 1 tablespoon lime juice (15ml)
- 1/32 teaspoon liquid stevia (or to taste)
- Fresh mint leaves for garnish

Instructions:

1. Arrange the pineapple slices on a large plate.
2. Drizzle with lime juice and liquid stevia, adjusting the amount based on your desired sweetness.
3. Garnish with fresh mint leaves.
4. Serve immediately as a refreshing, low-fat dessert.

Kcal: 75, Cho: 18g, Fat: 0g, Na: 0mg, Pro: 1g

Apple and Pear Crisp

Servings: 2

Prep Time: 10 minutes

Cook Time: 25 minutes

Ingredients:

- 1 apple, sliced (150g)
- 1 pear, sliced (150g)
- 2 tablespoons rolled oats (16g)
- 1 tablespoon almond flour (7g)
- 1/16 teaspoon liquid stevia (or to taste)
- 1/2 teaspoon ground cinnamon (1g)

Instructions:

1. Preheat the oven to 375°F (190°C).
2. Arrange the apple and pear slices in a baking dish.
3. In a small bowl, mix oats, almond flour, stevia, and cinnamon. Adjust the stevia amount based on your desired sweetness.
4. Sprinkle the oat mixture over the fruit.
5. Bake for 25 minutes or until the topping is golden and the fruit is tender.
6. Serve warm.

Kcal: 145, Cho: 32g, Fat: 2g, Na: 0mg, Pro: 2g

Banana Soft Serve

Servings: 2

Prep Time: 5 minutes

Cook Time: 0 minutes

Ingredients:

- 2 bananas, sliced and frozen (240g)
- 1 teaspoon vanilla extract (5ml)

Instructions:

1. Place frozen banana slices in a blender or food processor.
2. Add vanilla extract.
3. Blend until smooth and creamy.
4. Serve immediately as a healthy ice cream alternative.

Kcal: 105, Cho: 27g, Fat: 0g, Na: 1mg, Pro: 1g

Mango Pudding

Servings: 2

Prep Time: 10 minutes

Cook Time: 0 minutes

Ingredients:

- 1 cup mango, diced (165g)
- 1/2 cup coconut milk (120ml)
- 1 tablespoon chia seeds (12g)
- 1/16 teaspoon liquid stevia (or to taste)

Instructions:

1. Combine mango, coconut milk, chia seeds, and stevia in a blender.
2. Blend until smooth. Adjust the amount of stevia based on your desired sweetness.
3. Pour the mixture into serving bowls.
4. Refrigerate for at least 1 hour to set.
5. Serve chilled.

Kcal: 165, Cho: 28g, Fat: 6g, Na: 15mg, Pro: 2g

Raspberry Coconut Bars

Servings: 2

Prep Time: 10 minutes

Cook Time: 15 minutes

Ingredients:

- 1 cup raspberries (125g)
- 1/2 cup shredded coconut (40g)
- 1/4 cup almond flour (28g)
- 1/8 teaspoon liquid stevia (or to taste)
- 1 tablespoon coconut oil, melted (15ml)

Instructions:

1. Preheat the oven to 350°F (175°C).
2. In a bowl, mix raspberries, shredded coconut, almond flour, stevia, and melted coconut oil. Adjust the stevia amount based on your desired sweetness.
3. Press the mixture into a small baking dish lined with parchment paper.
4. Bake for 15 minutes or until set and lightly golden.
5. Let cool before cutting into bars.
6. Serve as a tasty, low-fat treat.

Kcal: 195, Cho: 22g, Fat: 12g, Na: 10mg, Pro: 3g

Grilled Peaches with Stevia

Servings: 2

Prep Time: 5 minutes

Cook Time: 10 minutes

Ingredients:

- 2 peaches, halved and pitted (300g)
- 1/16 teaspoon liquid stevia (or to taste)
- 1/4 teaspoon ground cinnamon (1g)

Instructions:

1. Preheat grill to medium-high (375°F / 190°C).
2. Place peach halves on the grill, cut side down.
3. Grill for 4-5 minutes until grill marks appear.
4. Flip peaches and grill for another 4-5 minutes until tender.
5. Drizzle with liquid stevia, adjusting the amount to your desired sweetness, and sprinkle with cinnamon.
6. Serve warm.

Kcal: 105, Cho: 27g, Fat: 0g, Na: 0mg, Pro: 1g

Orange Chia Pudding

Servings: 2

Prep Time: 10 minutes

Cook Time: 0 minutes

Ingredients:

- 1 cup almond milk (240ml)
- 1/2 cup orange juice (120ml)
- 1/4 cup chia seeds (40g)
- 1/16 teaspoon liquid stevia (or to taste)
- 1/2 teaspoon vanilla extract (2ml)

Instructions:

1. In a bowl, mix almond milk, orange juice, chia seeds, stevia, and vanilla extract.
2. Stir well to combine. Adjust the amount of stevia based on your desired sweetness.
3. Refrigerate for at least 4 hours or overnight, stirring occasionally.
4. Serve chilled.

Kcal: 175, Cho: 24g, Fat: 8g, Na: 45mg, Pro: 4g

Berry Pavlova

Servings: 2

Prep Time: 15 minutes

Cook Time: 1 hour

Ingredients:

- 2 egg whites (60g)
- 1/2 cup sugar (100g)
- 1/4 teaspoon cream of tartar (1g)
- 1/2 teaspoon vanilla extract (2ml)
- 1/2 cup mixed berries (75g)

Instructions:

1. Preheat oven to 250°F (120°C). Line a baking sheet with parchment paper.
2. Beat egg whites and cream of tartar until soft peaks form.
3. Gradually add sugar, beating until stiff peaks form.
4. Fold in vanilla extract.

5. Spoon meringue onto the baking sheet, forming two small nests.
6. Bake for 1 hour, then turn off the oven and let meringues cool completely inside.
7. Top with mixed berries and serve.

Kcal: 150, Cho: 35g, Fat: 0g, Na: 35mg, Pro: 3g

Lemon Sorbet

Servings: 2

Prep Time: 10 minutes

Cook Time: 0 minutes

Ingredients:

- 1 cup water (240ml)
- 1/2 cup sugar (100g)
- 1/2 cup lemon juice (120ml)
- 1 teaspoon lemon zest (2g)

Instructions:

1. In a saucepan, combine water and sugar. Heat until sugar dissolves.
2. Remove from heat and stir in lemon juice and zest.
3. Pour the mixture into a freezer-safe container.
4. Freeze for 4-6 hours, stirring occasionally.
5. Scoop into bowls and serve.

Kcal: 120, Cho: 30g, Fat: 0g, Na: 0mg, Pro: 0g

Watermelon Pizza

Servings: 2

Prep Time: 10 minutes

Cook Time: 0 minutes

Ingredients:

- 1 large slice of watermelon (300g)
- 1/2 cup Greek yogurt (low-fat) (120g)
- 1/4 cup blueberries (37g)
- 1/4 cup strawberries, sliced (37g)
- 1/16 teaspoon liquid stevia (or to taste)
- Fresh mint leaves for garnish

Instructions:

1. Spread Greek yogurt over the watermelon slice.
2. Top with blueberries and sliced strawberries.
3. Drizzle with liquid stevia, adjusting the amount to your desired sweetness.
4. Garnish with fresh mint leaves.
5. Cut into wedges and serve immediately.

Kcal: 140, Cho: 27g, Fat: 2g, Na: 30mg, Pro: 6g

Kiwi and Strawberry Layered Gelatin

Servings: 2

Prep Time: 15 minutes

Cook Time: 0 minutes

Ingredients:

- 1 cup boiling water (240ml)
- 1 packet unflavored gelatin (7g)
- 1 cup cold water (240ml)
- 1/2 cup kiwi, diced (75g)
- 1/2 cup strawberries, sliced (75g)
- 1/16 teaspoon liquid stevia (or to taste)

Instructions:

1. Dissolve gelatin in boiling water, then add cold water and stevia. Stir well. Adjust the amount of stevia based on your desired sweetness.
2. Pour half of the gelatin mixture into serving glasses and add kiwi.
3. Refrigerate for 1 hour until set.
4. Add the remaining gelatin mixture and layer with strawberries.
5. Refrigerate for another hour until fully set.
6. Serve chilled.

Kcal: 50, Cho: 13g, Fat: 0g, Na: 10mg, Pro: 2g

Poached Pears with Cinnamon

Servings: 2

Prep Time: 5 minutes

Cook Time: 20 minutes

Ingredients:

- 2 pears, peeled and halved (300g)
- 2 cups water (480ml)
- 1/8 teaspoon liquid stevia (or to taste)
- 1 cinnamon stick

Instructions:

1. In a saucepan, bring water, stevia, and the cinnamon stick to a boil. Adjust the amount of stevia based on your desired sweetness.
2. Reduce heat to low and add pear halves.
3. Simmer for 20 minutes until pears are tender.
4. Remove pears and let cool slightly.
5. Serve warm or chilled.

Kcal: 85, Cho: 22g, Fat: 0g, Na: 0mg, Pro: 1g

Baked Grapefruit with Stevia and Mint

Servings: 2

Prep Time: 5 minutes

Cook Time: 15 minutes

Ingredients:

- 1 large grapefruit, halved (300g)
- 1/16 teaspoon liquid stevia (or to taste)
- Fresh mint leaves for garnish

Instructions:

1. Preheat oven to 375°F (190°C).
2. Place grapefruit halves on a baking sheet.
3. Drizzle each half with liquid stevia, adjusting the amount based on your desired sweetness.
4. Bake for 15 minutes until slightly caramelized.
5. Garnish with fresh mint leaves and serve warm.

Kcal: 60, Cho: 15g, Fat: 0g, Na: 0mg, Pro: 1g

Coconut Water Popsicles

Servings: 2

Prep Time: 10 minutes

Cook Time: 0 minutes

Ingredients:

- 1 cup coconut water (240ml)
- 1/2 cup mixed berries (75g)
- 1/16 teaspoon liquid stevia (or to taste)

Instructions:

1. In a bowl, mix coconut water and stevia until well combined. Adjust the amount of stevia based on your desired sweetness.
2. Divide mixed berries between popsicle molds.
3. Pour the coconut water mixture over the berries.
4. Insert sticks and freeze for at least 4 hours.
5. Serve frozen for a refreshing treat.

Kcal: 50, Cho: 12g, Fat: 0g, Na: 30mg, Pro: 1g

Pomegranate and Pistachio Dark Chocolate Bark

Servings: 2

Prep Time: 10 minutes

Cook Time: 10 minutes

Ingredients:

- 3.5 oz dark chocolate (100g)
- 1/4 cup pomegranate seeds (40g)
- 1/4 cup pistachios, chopped (30g)

Instructions:

1. Melt dark chocolate in a double boiler or microwave until smooth.
2. Pour melted chocolate onto a parchment-lined baking sheet, spreading it evenly.
3. Sprinkle pomegranate seeds and chopped pistachios over the chocolate.
4. Refrigerate for 1 hour until set.
5. Break into pieces and serve.

Kcal: 180, Cho: 20g, Fat: 10g, Na: 5mg, Pro: 3g

Chapter 11: 4-Week Kickstart Meal Plan

Week 1

Day	Breakfast	Lunch	Snack	Dinner	Dessert

Monday	Cinnamon Apple Yogurt Parfait	Grilled Veggie and Hummus Wrap	Greek Yogurt and Mixed Berries	Vegetable Stir Fry with Tofu	Raspberry Coconut Bars
Tuesday	Savory Oatmeal with Avocado	Chicken Salad with Mixed Greens	Carrot and Hummus Dip	Turkey Meatballs with Zucchini Noodles	Pineapple Carpaccio
Wednesday	Banana Pancakes	Broccoli and Cauliflower Soup	Spiced Pumpkin Seeds	Herb-Roasted Chicken Breast	Mango Pudding
Thursday	Egg White Scramble with Spinach	Cauliflower Rice Burrito Bowl	Almond Butter Apple Slices	Grilled Eggplant with Tomato Salad	Pomegranate and Pistachio Dark Chocolate Bark
Friday	Sunrise Smoothie Bowl	Asian Chicken Salad	Roasted Chickpeas	Veggie-Packed Paella	Chocolate Avocado Mousse
Saturday	Apple Cinnamon Porridge	Zucchini Noodles with Pesto	Avocado Egg Salad	Coconut Curry with Chickpeas	Watermelon Pizza
Sunday	Multigrain Waffles	Stuffed Bell Peppers	Peanut Butter Banana Smoothie	Slow Cooker Pulled Chicken	Poached Pears with Cinnamon

Week 2

Day	Breakfast	Lunch	Snack	Dinner	Dessert
Monday	Berry Blast Overnight Oats	Spiced Lentil Tacos	Watermelon Mint Salad	Baked Salmon with Asparagus	Mixed Berry Sorbet
Tuesday	Spinach and Mushroom Egg Muffins	Turkey Lettuce Wrap	Beet and Carrot Juice	Spaghetti Squash with Marinara Sauce	Strawberry Cheesecake Cups
Wednesday	Tomato Basil Omelet	Butternut Squash Soup	Coconut Yogurt Parfait	Moroccan Vegetable Tagine	Baked Apples with Cinnamon

Thursday	Peach and Chia Pudding	Quinoa and Black Bean Salad	Pomegranate Blueberry Blast Smoothie	Cauliflower Steak with Olive Relish	Apple and Pear Crisp
Friday	Cottage Cheese and Pineapple Plate	Avocado Tuna Salad	Celery and Almond Butter	Beef and Broccoli Stir Fry	Peach Frozen Yogurt
Saturday	Green Tea Smoothie	Spicy Shrimp Stir Fry	Kale Chips	Grilled Portobello Mushrooms	Banana Soft Serve
Sunday	Banana Pancakes	Chicken Salad with Mixed Greens	Caprese Salad Skewers	Lemon Garlic Shrimp Skewers	Kiwi and Strawberry Layered Gelatin

Week 3

Day	Breakfast	Lunch	Snack	Dinner	Dessert
Monday	Almond and Banana Smoothie	Butternut Squash Soup	Berry and Spinach Smoothie	Herb-Roasted Chicken Breast	Berry Pavlova
Tuesday	Multigrain Waffles	Chicken and Veggie Kabobs	Air-Popped Popcorn with Sea Salt	Grilled Eggplant with Tomato Salad	Orange Chia Pudding
Wednesday	Cinnamon Apple Yogurt Parfait	Eggplant and Tomato Stew	Avocado Egg Salad	Pork Tenderloin with Roasted Apples	Coconut Water Popsicles
Thursday	Berry Quinoa Breakfast Bowl	Spinach and Strawberry Salad	Celery and Almond Butter	Grilled Tilapia with Mango Salsa	Poached Pears with Cinnamon
Friday	Savory Oatmeal with Avocado	Cauliflower Rice Burrito Bowl	Roasted Chickpeas	Ratatouille	Raspberry Coconut Bars
Saturday	Southwest Tofu Scramble	Turkey Lettuce Wraps	Mango Lime Smoothie	Roast Turkey with Cranberry Sauce	Lemon Sorbet

| Sunday | Pumpkin Spice Latte Smoothie | Chicken Salad with Mixed Greens | Carrot and Hummus Dip | Stuffed Acorn Squash | Grilled Peaches with Stevia |

Week 4

Day	Breakfast	Lunch	Snack	Dinner	Dessert
Monday	Multigrain Waffles	Zucchini Noodles with Pesto	Green Detox Smoothie	Veggie-Packed Paella	Apple and Pear Crisp
Tuesday	Tomato Basil Omelet	Grilled Veggie and Hummus Wrap	Cucumber Tomato Salad	Spaghetti Squash with Marinara Sauce	Kiwi and Strawberry Layered Gelatin
Wednesday	Peach and Chia Pudding	Broccoli and Cauliflower Soup	Coconut Yogurt Parfait	Beef and Broccoli Stir Fry	Chocolate Avocado Mousse
Thursday	Veggie-Packed Breakfast Burrito	Greek Salad with Chicken	Kale Chips	Cauliflower Steak with Olive Relish	Baked Apples with Cinnamon
Friday	Cinnamon Apple Yogurt Parfait	Spicy Shrimp Stir Fry	Caprese Salad Skewers	Lemon Garlic Shrimp Skewers	Watermelon Pizza
Saturday	Egg White Scramble with Spinach	Veggie and Lentil Soup	Spiced Pumpkin Seeds	Coconut Curry with Chickpeas	Peach Frozen Yogur
Sunday	Sunrise Smoothie Bowl	Curried Veggie Wrap	Watermelon Mint Salad	Baked Salmon with Asparagus	Mixed Berry Sorbet

Tips for Staying on Track

Plan Ahead

Planning your meals in advance can save time and help you stay committed to your goals. Having a weekly menu means you won't be caught off guard, reducing the temptation to opt for less healthy choices.

Keep Your Kitchen Stocked

Ensure your pantry and refrigerator are always stocked with the basics. Fresh fruits, vegetables, lean proteins, and whole grains should be readily available. This makes it easier to whip up a healthy meal at any time.

Stay Hydrated

Drinking enough water is crucial for overall health and can also help manage hunger. Sometimes our bodies mistake thirst for hunger, leading to unnecessary snacking.

Find a Buddy

Having a friend or family member join you in your healthy eating plan can provide motivation and accountability. Share recipes, cook together, or just check in with each other to stay on track.

Listen to Your Body

It's important to pay attention to your body's hunger and fullness cues. Eat when you're hungry and stop when you're satisfied, not stuffed. This helps in maintaining a healthy relationship with food.

Allow Flexibility

While it's good to have a plan, it's also important to be flexible. Life can be unpredictable, and sometimes plans change. Don't be too hard on yourself if you deviate from the plan occasionally. Just get back on track with your next meal.

Enjoy the Process

Cooking and eating should be enjoyable. Experiment with new recipes, savor the flavors, and appreciate the nourishment you're providing your body. Enjoying your meals makes it easier to stick to your healthy eating plan.

By following this structured plan and incorporating these tips, you'll be well on your way to mastering zero-point cooking and enjoying a healthier lifestyle. Happy cooking!

Chapter 12: Beyond the Diet

Maintaining the Zero Point Lifestyle Long-Term

Adopting the Zero Point Lifestyle is more than just following a diet; it's about making sustainable changes that support long-term health and wellness. To maintain this lifestyle effectively, it's crucial to integrate the principles of Zero Point eating into your daily routine seamlessly. Start by keeping your kitchen well-stocked with the basics: fresh fruits, vegetables, lean proteins, and whole grains. These staples will make it easier to prepare healthy meals without feeling deprived.

It's also essential to continue planning your meals. Regular meal planning helps prevent last-minute unhealthy choices and ensures you have the ingredients you need on hand. Consider dedicating a specific day each week to plan your meals and do your grocery shopping. This habit not only saves time but also reinforces your commitment to your health goals.

Another key aspect of maintaining the Zero Point Lifestyle is staying active. Regular physical activity complements healthy eating and enhances overall well-being. Find activities you enjoy, whether it's walking, cycling, swimming, or practicing yoga. Incorporate exercise into your daily routine, and remember that consistency is more important than intensity. Even small amounts of physical activity can make a significant difference when done regularly.

Listening to your body is vital. Pay attention to hunger and fullness cues, and eat mindfully. This means savoring each bite, eating slowly, and stopping when you feel satisfied, not stuffed. Mindful eating helps you appreciate the flavors and textures of your food and can prevent overeating.

Surround yourself with a supportive community. Whether it's friends, family, or an online group, having people who share your goals and encourage you can make a big difference. Share recipes, celebrate successes, and support each other through challenges. Social support can provide motivation and accountability, helping you stay on track.

Finally, be patient with yourself. Long-term change takes time, and it's normal to experience ups and downs. If you encounter setbacks, don't be too hard on yourself. Instead, focus on the progress you've made and recommit to your goals. Remember that maintaining a healthy lifestyle is a lifelong process, and every small step you take brings you closer to your goals.

Adjusting for Special Situations (Eating Out, Holidays)

Eating out and holidays can present unique challenges when trying to maintain the Zero Point Lifestyle, but with a little planning and mindfulness, you can navigate these situations successfully. When dining out, start by researching the menu in advance if possible. Many restaurants now provide nutritional information online, allowing you to make informed choices before you even arrive. Look for dishes that feature plenty of vegetables, lean proteins, and whole grains. Avoid items that are fried or covered in heavy sauces, as these can add unnecessary calories and fats.

Don't be afraid to ask for modifications to your meal. Most restaurants are happy to accommodate special requests, such as grilling instead of frying or serving dressings and sauces on the side. This way, you can control the amount you consume and make your meal healthier. Additionally, consider portion sizes. Restaurant portions are often much larger than what you would typically eat at home. You can request a half-portion, share a dish with a dining companion, or ask for a to-go box and save half for later.

When attending holiday gatherings, it's helpful to bring a dish that aligns with your dietary goals. This ensures there's at least one healthy option available and can also introduce others to the delicious possibilities of Zero Point eating. Focus on filling your plate with vegetables, fruits, and lean proteins, and enjoy treats in moderation. It's important to enjoy the social and cultural aspects of holiday meals without feeling guilty.

Practice mindful eating during these special occasions. Pay attention to what you're eating, savor each bite, and listen to your body's signals. This can help you avoid overeating and make more satisfying choices. Remember that it's okay to indulge occasionally. The key is to do so mindfully and get back to your usual eating habits afterward.

Staying active during holidays and special occasions can also help balance out any indulgences. Plan for a family walk after a big meal or engage in festive activities that involve physical movement. This not only helps manage your weight but also enhances your overall holiday experience.

When You Slip: Getting Back on Track

Everyone slips up from time to time, and that's perfectly normal. What's important is how you respond to these moments. The first step is to avoid the all-or-nothing mindset. Just because you've had a setback doesn't mean you've failed. Recognize that setbacks are a natural part of any long-term change and use them as learning opportunities.

Reflect on what led to the slip-up. Were you stressed, bored, or in a social situation where healthy options were limited? Understanding the triggers can help you develop strategies to manage them in the future. For example, if stress is a trigger, you might explore stress-relief techniques such as exercise, meditation, or talking to a friend.

Recommit to your goals by reminding yourself why you started the Zero Point Lifestyle in the first place. Think about the benefits you've experienced, whether it's increased energy, better health markers, or simply feeling more confident in your food choices. Reaffirming your motivations can help reignite your commitment.

Plan your next meal. After a slip-up, it can be tempting to continue eating off-plan, but the best way to get back on track is to make your next meal a healthy one. Plan a balanced, nutritious meal that includes plenty of Zero Point foods. This helps reset your mindset and reinforces your commitment to your goals.

Seek support from your community. Share your experience with friends, family, or an online group. Not only can they offer encouragement and advice, but discussing your challenges openly can also help you feel less isolated. Remember that everyone faces setbacks, and sharing can foster a sense of solidarity and mutual support.

Finally, practice self-compassion. Be kind to yourself and recognize that making lasting changes takes time and effort. Celebrate your progress, no matter how small, and focus on moving forward. Each day is a new opportunity to make healthy choices and continue your journey toward better health.

Incorporating these strategies into your lifestyle can help you maintain the Zero Point Lifestyle long-term, navigate special situations with confidence, and recover quickly from any setbacks. Remember that the key to success is consistency, mindfulness, and a positive attitude. By making these principles a part of your everyday life, you can enjoy the benefits of a healthy, balanced diet and achieve your long-term health goals.

Conclusion

As we reach the end of this book, it's important to take a moment to reflect on the progress you've made. Transitioning to the Zero Point Lifestyle is a significant step towards a healthier, more balanced life. It's not just about losing weight; it's about cultivating a sustainable relationship with food that nourishes both body and mind.

Think back to when you first started. Perhaps you felt overwhelmed by the idea of changing your eating habits. You might have doubted whether you could stick to the plan or worried about missing out on your favorite foods. Reflect on how far you've come since then. You've discovered new recipes, explored different flavors, and learned to appreciate the natural tastes of wholesome ingredients. Each step, no matter how small, has contributed to your progress.

The recipes and meal plans provided here have hopefully made the transition smoother and more enjoyable. Cooking and eating should be pleasurable activities, and the Zero Point Lifestyle aims to keep it that way. By focusing on nutrient-dense, low-calorie foods, you've given yourself the freedom to enjoy satisfying meals without the constant stress of calorie counting.

Reflecting on your progress also means acknowledging the challenges you've faced. Maybe there were days when you strayed from the plan or felt tempted by less healthy options. These moments are part of the process. They provide valuable lessons and help you build resilience. By understanding your triggers and learning how to navigate them, you become better equipped to maintain your healthy habits in the long run.

Future Steps and Continuous Improvement

Looking ahead, it's essential to keep the momentum going. The Zero Point Lifestyle is not a temporary diet but a long-term commitment to your well-being. Continuous improvement is key. As you become more comfortable with this way of eating, consider expanding your culinary horizons even further.

Start by experimenting with new ingredients and recipes. The world of healthy eating is vast and varied, offering endless possibilities for delicious meals. Try incorporating more plant-based options, exploring different cuisines, and using herbs and spices to enhance flavors. Cooking should be a creative and enjoyable process, so don't be afraid to step outside your comfort zone.

Additionally, keep educating yourself about nutrition. Understanding the science behind your food choices empowers you to make informed decisions. Stay updated with the latest research, attend workshops, or join online communities focused on healthy living. The more knowledge you gain, the better you can tailor the Zero Point Lifestyle to fit your personal needs and preferences.

Regularly reassess your goals. As you achieve milestones, set new ones to keep yourself motivated. These goals don't have to be solely about weight loss. They can include improving your cooking skills, increasing your physical activity, or even growing your own vegetables.

Celebrate your achievements, no matter how small, and use them as stepping stones for further progress.

It's also important to remain flexible and adapt to changes. Life is unpredictable, and there will be times when sticking to the plan becomes challenging. Whether it's due to a busy schedule, travel, or social events, remember that flexibility is key. Allow yourself the grace to deviate occasionally without feeling guilty. The goal is to cultivate a balanced lifestyle that you can maintain over the long term.

Thanks to Contributors and Supporters

No progress is ever undertaken alone, and your transition to the Zero Point Lifestyle is no exception. It's time to acknowledge and thank those who have supported you along the way. First and foremost, gratitude goes to the nutritionists and culinary experts who contributed their knowledge and expertise to this book. Their insights have provided a solid foundation for the recipes and meal plans that have guided you.

A heartfelt thanks to the farmers and food producers who work tirelessly to provide fresh, wholesome ingredients. Their dedication to sustainable and ethical farming practices ensures that we have access to the best quality produce. Supporting local and organic farms not only benefits your health but also contributes to a more sustainable food system.

To the friends and family members who have encouraged and supported you, your progress would not have been the same without them. Their understanding and encouragement have been invaluable, whether through sharing meals, offering words of encouragement, or simply being there when you needed a boost.

Finally, a special thank you to you, the reader. Your commitment to improving your health and well-being is inspiring. By choosing the Zero Point Lifestyle, you are taking proactive steps towards a better future, not just for yourself but for those around you. Your determination and perseverance are commendable, and you should be proud of the progress you've made.

Final Words

As you continue on this path, remember that the road to a healthier lifestyle is a marathon, not a sprint. There will be ups and downs, moments of triumph, and times of struggle. The key is to stay focused on your goals and remain committed to the principles of the Zero Point Lifestyle.

Every meal is an opportunity to nourish your body and mind. Embrace the simplicity and joy of eating whole, natural foods. Celebrate the flavors, textures, and colors that nature provides. Cooking and eating should be acts of self-love and care, not burdens or obligations.

When challenges arise, remind yourself of why you started. Think about the positive changes you've experienced, whether it's increased energy, improved mood, or better overall health. Let these benefits serve as motivation to keep going.

Stay connected with your support network. Share your experiences, ask for advice, and offer encouragement to others. Together, we can create a community that thrives on mutual support and shared goals. Remember that you are never alone on this path.

Lastly, be kind to yourself. Perfection is not the goal; progress is. Celebrate your victories, learn from your setbacks, and keep moving forward. The Zero Point Lifestyle is about creating a sustainable, enjoyable way of eating that supports your long-term health and happiness.

As you move forward, carry with you the knowledge, skills, and confidence you've gained. Continue to explore, learn, and grow. The path to a healthier life is always evolving, and each step you take brings you closer to your goals.

Thank you for allowing this book to be a part of your progress. Here's to a future filled with delicious meals, vibrant health, and endless possibilities. Keep cooking, keep exploring, and most importantly, keep taking care of yourself. You've got this!

Made in United States
Orlando, FL
17 October 2024

52800520R00057